"During the last years we have seen an impressive development of the evidence base for music therapy. An important remaining challenge is to develop valid assessment tools that are sensitive to the specific changes that music therapy induces. John Carpente's new book helps to fill that gap by presenting a set of music-centered rating scales that examine clients' capacity to musically interact and thus present a musical way of thinking about, working with, and understanding clients. The author's previous involvement in developing improvisational music therapy for people with autism and his current involvement in the first international multicenter trial in the area (the TIME-A project) make it likely that this book and the scales presented therein will be widely used by clinicians and researchers."

Christian Gold, Ph.D.
Principal Researcher, GAMUT, Uni Research, Bergen, Norway
Professor, University of Bergen, Norway
Editor-in-Chief, *Nordic Journal of Music Therapy*

"With this publication of the IMCAP-ND assessment manual, Dr. Carpente provides an invaluable resource for music therapists who provide services to people with autism and other neurodevelopmental disorders. This clinical manual clearly defines and organizes specific music responses as they relate to interaction, communication, cognition and perception, and responsiveness. The IMCAP-ND includes three rating scales that are easily scored and compiled and which give solid information on the client's strengths and needs as well as clear guidance on setting clinical goals."

Elizabeth K. Schwartz, M.A., LCAT, MT-BC
Co-Founder, Raising Harmony: Music Therapy for Young Children
Senior Music Therapist, Alternatives for Children, Long Island, NY
Author: *Music, Therapy, and Early Childhood: A Developmental Approach*

"John Carpente is a gifted clinician and researcher, who, with this new publication, makes a significant contribution to the field of music therapy in the area of clinical assessment. He has carefully integrated theoretical concepts of Nordoff-Robbins Music Therapy with Greenspan's Developmental – Individual Differences – Relationship (DIR®) model and Floortime™ principles to create a unique music-centered assessment profiling tool for neurodiverse children. By 'following the client's musical emotional lead,' this assessment instrument promotes a respectful and accepting musical environment to assess clients' needs and strengths. This clinical manual will be an indispensable tool for all music therapists who believe in the power of affect to help clients relate and communicate through the experience of musical-play."

Cecilia Breinbauer, M.D.
Director, Interdisciplinary Council on Developmental and Learning Disorders (ICDL)

"The IMCAP-ND offers the music therapist a developmental and relational framework to understand, assess, and promote human development in those children and adults with neurodevelopmental profiles that render them less available for reciprocal relationships. Through the elements of musicality, Dr. Carpente offers three remarkable scales that reveal and strengthen emotional, cognitive, and relational capacities that cannot be assessed through traditional psychometric instruments. The IMCAP-ND adds to multidisciplinary, developmentally-driven ways to discern and strengthen human capacities. The 'right brain' is given voice in the IMCAP-ND and offers all pediatric disciplines a window into the full range of human drama."

Gerard Costa, Ph.D.
Director and Senior Lecturer, Center for Autism and Early Childhood Mental Health, College of Education and Human Services, Montclair State University

IMCAP-ND

The Individual Music-Centered Assessment Profile for Neurodevelopmental Disorders

IMCAP-ND

The Individual Music-Centered Assessment Profile for Neurodevelopmental Disorders

A Clinical Manual

John A. Carpente
Foreword by Brian Abrams

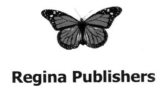

Regina Publishers

IMCAP-ND
The Individual Music-Centered Assessment Profile for Neurodevelopmental Disorders:
A Clinical Manual

Copyright © 2013 by John A. Carpente

All rights reserved.
No part of this book may be reproduced, stored in a retrieval system, or transmitted in any form, or by any means, electronic, mechanical, photocopying, recording or otherwise, without prior permission of the author.

ISBN-10: 0989179001
ISBN-13: 978-0-9891790-0-3

Distributed throughout the world by:
Regina Publishers
C/o Developmental Music Health
P.O. Box 1711
North Baldwin, NY 11510
www.DMHmusictherapy.com

Cover design by Francis Bonnet

In loving memory of my mother, Regina

TABLE OF CONTENTS

FOREWORD xiii

ACKNOWLEDGMENTS xvii

INTRODUCTION: OVERVIEW OF THE MANUAL 1
    Overview of Chapters 1
    Chapter 1 1
    Chapter 2 2
    Chapters 3, 4, and 5 2
        Scale I: Musical Emotional Assessment Rating Scale 2
        Scale II: Musical Cognitive/Perception Scale 3
        Scale III: Musical Responsiveness Scale 4

CHAPTER 1: OVERVIEW OF THE IMCAP-ND 5
    Summary of Chapter 5
    Description 5
    Data Collection 6
    Therapist's Qualifications 8
    Population-based 8

CHAPTER 2: GENERAL OUTLINE OF MUSIC THERAPY SESSIONS 11
    Summary of Chapter 11
    Session Format 11
    Musical Media 12
    Musical-Play 12
    Clinical Improvisation 13
    Clinical Techniques 14
    Procedural Considerations 15
    Procedural Phases 16
        Following the client's musical emotional lead 17
        Two-way purposeful music making 21
        Affect synchrony in musical-play 23
        Quality of musical-play interactions 24
        Range in musical-play 26
        Intentionality in musical-play 26

    Procedures for Supportive Interventions 28
        Minimal support 30
        Mild support 30
        Moderate support 32
        Maximum support 33

CHAPTER 3: SCALE I: MUSICAL EMOTIONAL ASSESSMENT RATING SCALE 35

    Summary of Chapter 35
    Musical Emotional Assessment Rating Scale (MEARS) 35
    Level I: Musical Attention 36
    Assessing Musical Attention 36
        Instructions 36
        Clinical techniques 38
        Considerations 38
    Level II: Musical Affect 39
    Assessing Musical Affect 40
        Instructions 40
        Clinical techniques 41
        Considerations 41
    Level III: Adaption to Musical-Play 42
    Assessing Adaption to Musical-Play 42
        Instructions 42
        Clinical techniques 44
        Considerations 44
    Level IV: Musical Engagement 45
    Assessing Musical Engagement 46
        Instructions 46
        Clinical techniques 47
        Considerations 47
    Level V: Musical Interrelatedness 48
    Assessing Musical Interrelatedness 49
        Instructions 49
        Clinical techniques 50
        Considerations 50
    Scoring Instructions 51
    Analyzing and Interpreting Scores 52

CHAPTER 4: SCALE II: MUSICAL COGNITIVE/PERCEPTION SCALE 55

Summary of Chapter 55
The Musical Cognitive/Perception Scale (MCPS) 55
Area I: Reacts 56
Observation and listening 56
Clinical techniques 57
Considerations 57
Area II: Focus 59
Observation and listening 59
Clinical techniques 60
Considerations 60
Area III: Recall 61
Observation and listening 61
Clinical techniques 62
Considerations 62
Area IV: Follow 63
Observation and listening 63
Clinical techniques 64
Considerations 64
Area V: Initiate 65
Observation and listening 65
Clinical techniques 66
Considerations 66
Scoring Instructions 67
Analyzing and Interpreting Scores 68

CHAPTER 5: SCALE III: MUSICAL RESPONSIVENESS SCALE 69

Summary of Chapter 69
The Musical Responsiveness Scale (MRS) 69
Area I: Preferences 70
Observation: Preferences/vocal 70
Observation: Preferences/instrument 71
Observation: Preferences/movement 72
Clinical techniques 72
Considerations 73

- Area II: Perceptual Efficiency 73
  - Observation: Perceptual efficiency/vocal 74
  - Observation: Perceptual efficiency/instrument 74
  - Observation: Perceptual efficiency/movement 75
  - Clinical techniques 76
  - Considerations 76
- Area III: Self-Regulation 77
  - Observation: Self-regulation/vocal 77
  - Observation: Self-regulation/instrument 78
  - Observation: Self-regulation/movement 79
  - Clinical techniques 79
  - Considerations 80
- Scoring Instructions 81
- Analyzing and Interpreting Scores 82

GLOSSARY 85
APPENDIX A 89
IMCAP-ND FORMS 89
- Intake Form 91
- Rating Scales 101
- Assessment/Evaluation Report 111

REFERENCES 121
ABOUT THE AUTHOR 125
SUBJECT INDEX 127

FOREWORD

Some dream; some actually get things done. Dr. John Carpente is one of those rare individuals who *gets dreams done*. A no-nonsense, down-to-earth New Yorker and lifelong musician, he has brought both his innate talents as an artist and his tireless supply of empathy, playfulness, and joy to his work with a wide variety of clients (primarily children) to his distinguished career as a model music therapy clinician and scholar. His gifts to humankind have been numerous, not the least of which has been the founding of the internationally renowned Rebecca Center for Music Therapy. Driven by his own passion and recognition of the public need for a music-centered, relationship-based understanding of music therapy, John has constructed—through unflagging labors and consistent openness to mentor and peer input—the foundations of a music therapy assessment model documented in the present manual: *The Individual Music-Centered Assessment Profile for Neurodevelopmental Disorders (IMCAP-ND)*.

Neurodevelopmental disorders (a general category that includes autism spectrum disorders, Williams syndrome, ADD-HD, and so forth) have vexed health care professionals for centuries. Etiologies of these disorders have been attributed to numerous environmental, psycho-emotional, chemical, and genetic factors, accompanied by prescribed treatments based accordingly upon the presumed causes. The best, most recent evidence suggests that neurodevelopmental disorders are rooted within a particular "family" of forms of architecture and/or chemistry within the central nervous system, resulting in atypical sensory processes and emotional experiences, and manifesting as certain characteristic developmental progressions during childhood. These, in turn, constitute atypical patterns of *relating to others*—often in ways that present major challenges to a person's everyday experience of life, to dynamics involving family or other primary caregivers, and to adjustment in social and academic areas.

Over the years, as the legitimacy of communities consisting of persons diagnosed with neurodevelopmental disorders has begun to receive public acknowledgment, the notion that these atypical ways of experiencing the world should even be considered "disorders" has been challenged. Nonetheless, there is still general agreement that their associated circumstances present a distinct set of obstacles to functioning, and to actualization of individual, human potential. In spite of some relatively new pharmacological treatments that have been tested and utilized, no definitive medical intervention thus far exists. However, various therapeutic approaches for helping to improve opportunities for persons with neurodevelopmental disorders have emerged. Some of these approaches have emphasized modifying components of behavior via skillful stimulus-response patterns as the central purpose of therapy. Others have focused upon developing new possibilities for relating and for experiencing relationship on the level of individualized, human identity. The IMCAP-ND is an embodiment of the latter approach, constituting a music therapy assessment seated squarely within the greater continuum of individualized, relationship-oriented therapies.

In the IMCAP-ND, John has ingeniously formulated a way to assess clients in the manner most congruent with the very modality through which the work takes place: the music. The methodically crafted model anchors the often ineffable, relational experiences embodied within the extemporaneous *musicking* between client and therapist in a series of developmentally based, quantitative scales. At each level, and throughout every facet of the instrument, the role of creative play remains front and center. Music is not relegated to a separate "domain"—rather, it is understood as the experience and act of developmental, relational functioning that is the core basis for the client's initial referral to therapy (i.e., problems with intentional, spontaneous, affective, interactive relating). The model provides not only measures for administering the assessment for the purposes of measurement along the various continua of concern, but also a set of guiding principles for conducting the therapeutic work inextricable from the assessment process. In essence, it is a guide for doing quality music therapy, and therefore intrinsically challenges the musical, interpersonal, and clinical integrity of the assessor's skills.

In the IMCAP-ND, music is treated as something that happens by, for, and between people, and as something that is simultaneously the *means* through which a client's possibilities for relating grows, and the *end* or *goal* in therapy, based upon an understanding of music as something that embodies and expresses in one of the most (if not *the* most) comprehensively relational human domains. According to the theoretical underpinnings of the model, a shift in a client's way of relating within the music is, already, a clear and undeniable evidential shift in that client's way of relating in life. Unlike anything previously witnessed within the history of music therapy, the IMCAP-ND grounds this evidence of human transformation within a systematic framework that can effectively transfer in relevant ways across a diversity of health disciplines.

The IMCAP-ND stands upon the shoulders of the prior works of numerous giants who inhabit a pantheon of play-oriented and relationship-oriented neurodevelopmental theorist/practitioners, such as Stanley Greenspan, founder of the DIR®/Floortime™ model, and Paul Nordoff and Clive Robbins, founders of the Nordoff-Robbins Music Therapy model. Major contributions also include the developmental theory of Jean Piaget and the taxonomic classification of improvisational music therapy techniques by Ken Bruscia. The unparalleled virtues in the work of these figures bear witness to the greatness of what John has created in his model.

The IMCAP-ND is a paradigm shift and revolutionary force and will surely transform the very landscape of music therapy assessment. Without question, it will find its way into the modus operandi of music therapy professionals worldwide who work with people living with neurodevelopmental disorders, who are conducting research in this area, and/or who serve as clinical supervisors or instructors for students learning about this work, all while helping—through its remarkably transparent and accessible nature—to continue building professional bridges with disciplines outside of music therapy. Beyond this, it will rock the very foundations of how the music therapy field, and the public in general, has come to understand people living with neurodevelopmental disorders, as well as the role of music in working them.

It is my sincere belief that we owe John our heartfelt gratitude for his tireless persistence and generosity represented in his gift of this model, which will surely play a pivotal role in making the world a better place. We should applaud him for his efforts, and acknowledge him for his undeniable love for the music therapy field and for humanity. I, for one, thank him for getting this dream done.

Brian Abrams, Ph.D., MT-BC
Coordinator of Music Therapy
Montclair State University
March 2013

Acknowledgments

I would like to express my gratitude to the many people who saw me through this book; to all those who provided support, talked things over, and offered comments. To my colleagues at The Rebecca Center for Music Therapy at Molloy College—Jill Lucente, Gabriela Ortiz, Midori Osorto, and Suzanne Sorel—I thank you for your thought-provoking questions, encouragement, and contributions throughout the development of this book.

To Kenneth Bruscia, my mentor and friend, I can't thank you enough for your teachings, writings, guidance, insights, and challenging questions. You have influenced my practice, writing, and thinking in more ways than you can ever imagine.

Also, to my good friend and colleague Brian Abrams, I thank you for your friendship, encouragement, perspective, and for all of the rich discussions throughout the unfolding of this book.

To Cheryl Dileo, I thank you for your teachings, sincere support, and continuous encouragement throughout the years.

To my teachers from the days of my Nordoff-Robbins training in New York—Kenneth Aigen, Michele Ritholz, and Alan Turry—I thank you for introducing me to the guiding principles that continue to steer my music therapy work. A special thank you must go to the late great Clive Robbins for passionately expanding my perspective and understanding of the therapeutic potential and value of music. It was an honor to experience your humanity, spirit, passion, creativity, and knowledge. Your "being" will forever inspire and be a part of me.

To the late Stanley I. Greenspan, co-creator of the DIR®/Floortime™ model, I thank you for insurmountably influencing my thinking as a therapist, and as a parent. It was a privilege to be a part of your weekly supervision talks and I cannot imagine my work today without referring to your brilliance.

To my colleagues in the Music Therapy Department at Molloy College—Jesse Asch, Lora Heller, Seung-A Kim, and Evelyn Selesky—I thank you for your support, encouragement, and flexibility.

To my in-laws, Willie and Maria Kern I thank you for your love, support, and willingness to always be there to lend a helping hand.

To my dad Santiago, sister Genevieve, and uncle Jake, I thank each of you for your love and support throughout my music and music therapy careers. And to my late mother, Regina Carpente, I dedicate this book to you. You have been and will always be my hero. You brought music into my being and made sure that I was nourished with an assortment of life's treasures. You are forever in my heart.

To my loving wife, Susan, and two beautiful children, Olivia and Jason, I thank you for your patience, support, love, and for allowing me to pursue my passions.

And finally, to my greatest teachers, the children, who I have had the privilege of *musicking* with; I thank you all for your life lessons, expanding my music, and for allowing me to be a part of your musical journey.

INTRODUCTION: OVERVIEW OF THE MANUAL

The Individual Music-Centered Assessment Profile for Neurodevelopmental Disorders (IMCAP-ND) is a criterion-referenced assessment of musical interaction, communication, cognition and perception, and responsiveness in musical-play for individuals with neurodevelopmental disorders. The IMCAP-ND can be used to evaluate clients at various developmental levels and chronological ages from children to adults.

Administering the IMCAP-ND requires the therapist to improvise music experiences based on the client's interests and musical lead, while targeting specific musical responses that are relevant to neurodevelopmental disorders. The IMCAP-ND examines musical-emotional abilities, musical cognition and perception skills, as well as musical responsiveness that deals with preferences, perceptual efficiency, and self-regulation in musical-play.

Overview of the Chapters

The IMCAP-ND manual was designed to provide music therapists with a method to assess and evaluate a client's musical resources, strengths, challenges, and overall responsiveness (i.e., preference, efficiency, and self-regulation) in musical-play. The IMCAP-ND manual includes three interrelated rating scales, operational definitions and criteria of target responses, assessment protocols, musical-clinical and interpersonal procedures, instructions for clinical observation and listening, procedures for supportive interventions, clinical considerations, and descriptions and rationale for clinical strategies and techniques.

Chapter 1

Chapter 1 provides the therapist with an introduction to the IMCAP-ND including its purpose and function, the data collection process, therapist's qualifications, as well as a summary of neurodevelopmental disorders.

Chapter 2

Chapter 2 details the session format, description of media used in session, definition of musical-play and clinical improvisation, and presents clinical techniques that are specific to the IMCAP-ND. In addition, the chapter discusses procedural considerations, three working phases within the process of musical interaction, range and intentionality in musical-play, and evaluating quality in musical-play interactions. Furthermore, the chapter offers procedures for dealing with perseverative behaviors in musical-play and outlines protocols and criteria for implementing supportive interventions.

Chapters 3, 4, and 5

Chapters 3, 4, and 5 provide detailed descriptions of the three rating scales that make up the IMCAP-ND—Scale I: Musical Emotional Assessment Rating Scale (MEARS), Scale II: Musical Cognitive/Perception Scale (MCPS), and Scale III: Musical Responsiveness Scale (MRS).

The three scales, collectively, are designed to evaluate and identify the client's musical resources, challenges, strengths, preferences, and overall responsiveness. Scale II (MCPS) (Chapter 4) and Scale III (MRS) (Chapter 5) provide the therapist with the client's musical cognitive and perception abilities, preferences, and tendencies in musical-play, while Scale I (MEARS) examines the client's social-emotional capacities in musical-play, i.e., attending, responding affectively, adapting, engaging, and interrelating.

Scale I: Musical Emotional Assessment Rating Scale

The Musical Emotional Assessment Rating Scale (MEARS) described in Chapter 3 is a criterion-referenced rating scale designed to examine the client's musical ability to attend, respond affectively, adapt/engage in parallel play, engage/participate in parallel-interactive play, and interrelate/engage in true interactive play (see Figure 1). The MEARS is based on five specific music domain areas: 1) *musical attention,* 2) *musical-affect,* 3) *adaption to musical-play,* 4) *musical engagement,* and 5) *musical interrelatedness.* Scoring the MEARS is based on the frequency of target response, level of support provided for the target response, as well as indicating the media in which the client offered the response. Chapter 3 discusses the scale in detail, including the sequence and criteria of each music domain area, clinical protocols and procedures, techniques, considerations, and scoring protocols.

Figure 1. Example of MEARS

I. MUSICAL ATTENTION			
	Frequency	Support	Media
a) Focuses	3	4	I,V
b) Maintains	3	4	I,V
c) Shares	1	3	I,V,M
d) Shifts	1	3	I
Totals/Avg.	8/2	14/3.5	I,V,M

Scale II: Musical Cognitive/Perception Scale

Chapter 4 presents the Musical Cognitive/Perception Scale (MCPS), a criterion-referenced scale designed to examine the client's ability to react, focus, recall, follow, and initiate five musical elements, i.e., rhythm, melody, dynamic, phrase, and timbre. Scoring the MCPS is based on the frequency of the target response as well as indicating the media in which the client offered the response. Chapter 4 discusses the framework of the MCPS and defines each construct of the scale (see Figure 2). Chapter 4 also provides detailed descriptions of the clinical protocols, operational definitions and criteria for each target response, procedures, techniques, considerations, and scoring protocols.

Figure 2. Example of the MCPS

	Rhythm	Melody	Dynamic	Phrase	Timbre	Total/ Avg.
Reacts	I/4; M/4	V/5; M/5	I/2; V/2	V/2	V/2	26/3.25
Focuses	I/4	V/2	I/3; V/2	I/4	V/4; I/3	22/3.14
Recalls	I/2	I/2; V/1	M/3; I/4	V/2; I/3	V/3; I/2	22/2.44
Follows	I/1; M/1	1	I/2	1	V/1; I/1	8/1.14
Initiates	1	1	I/1; V/1	1	1	6/1.00

Scale III: Musical Responsiveness Scale

The Musical Responsiveness Scale (MRS), introduced in chapter 5, is a criterion-based rating scale designed to evaluate the client's overall responsiveness and tendencies in musical-play. Hence, the MRS deals with examining the client's musical preferences, perceptual efficiency, and ability to self-regulate in musical-play (see Figure 3). Scoring is based on the frequency of the target response in each media, i.e., vocal, instrumental, and movement. In addition, the chapter also discusses and operationally defines each construct of the scale, provides criteria for each target response, clinical procedures, techniques, considerations, and scoring protocols.

Figure 3. Example of the MRS

		TEMPO RANGE			DYN. RANGE			PITCH RANGE			ATTACK		
		Slow	Med	Fast	Soft	Med	Loud	Low	Mid	High	PS	SL	PL
V O C A L	Preference	1	1	1	3	1	3	1	3	1	3	1	1
	Efficiency	1	1	1	3	1	3	1	3	1	3	1	1
	Self-Regulation	1-	1-	1-	3	1-	3	1-	3	1-	3	1	1

CHAPTER 1 OVERVIEW OF THE IMCAP-ND

Summary of the Chapter

This chapter provides an overview of the IMCAP-ND, including defining its function and purpose as well as introducing all of its components and the three rating scales (MEARS, MCPS, and MRS). The chapter also describes data sources, the data collection process, and therapist qualifications. In addition, the chapter closes with briefly discussing the IMCAP-ND as a population-based assessment specific to neurodevelopmental disorders.

Description

The Individual Music-Centered Assessment Profile for Neurodevelopmental Disorders (IMCAP-ND) is a method for observing, listening, and rating musical emotional responses, cognition and perception, and preferences and efficiency in individuals diagnosed with neurodevelopmental disorders. Overall the IMCAP-ND focuses on how a client perceives, interprets, and creates music with the therapist as the first step in formulating goals and strategies for clinically working with the client. To administer the IMCAP-ND, the therapist improvises music experiences to engage the individual in target musical responses that are relevant to neurodevelopmental disorders. The IMCAP-ND may be completed by an observer during the session, or by the therapist immediately at the end of the session. The session may also be video-recorded and completed later by either observer or therapist; however, this is not necessary.

The IMCAP-ND consists of three rating scales. They include: 1) Scale I: Musical Emotional Assessment Rating Scale (MEARS) (Chapter 3), 2) Scale II: Musical Cognitive/Perception Scale (MCPS) (Chapter 4), and 3) Scale III: Musical Responsiveness Scale (MRS) (Chapter 5). Each scale can be completed in ten to fifteen minutes each, for a total of forty-five minutes.

The main purpose of the IMCAP-ND is to identify musical resources, needs, and preferences of an individual with neurodevelopmental disorders. This information in turn is used to guide the therapist in working with the client, as well as to inform others working with the client on his/her therapeutic and personal resources and needs. In addition, the rating scales can be used as pre- and posttest measures to evaluate client progress, on either a short- or long-term basis.

Data Collection

Sources of data for the IMCAP-ND are historical records, client–therapist musical interactions, and clinical observations. The first step of the assessment process is to collect historical data and caregiver reports of current functioning. This may include reports from the client's other therapists and educators. The purpose of examining the reports is to note any factors that may inform the IMCAP-ND assessment process.

When administering the IMCAP-ND, the therapist's main focus is on engaging the client in a wide variety of musical interactions, all within the context of play. Sessions may involve the client in playing instruments, singing, and/or moving. The media of playing, singing, and moving "are important because of the nature of the tasks and challenges contained within each experience" (Wheeler, Shultis, & Polen, 2005, p. 39). Thus, as the client participates in these music experiences, the therapist has an opportunity to assess what the client is able to perceive and do musically, and then engage the client in increasingly more challenging musical tasks until the client's musical resources and strengths can be clearly defined.

Clinical observations/listening then are the third source of data, and these observations may be made during or after the session by either the therapist conducting the session or by a trained observer.

The therapist may choose to observe the client through the course of one or several sessions. Sessions may be video-recorded although it is not required. If video-recording sessions is not an option, it is then required that the therapist score and take notes immediately following the session.

During each session the therapist improvises music based on the client's responses, reactions, and behaviors. Thus, observations are focused on how the client perceives, interprets, and creates music with the therapist. All aspects of the client's musical-play must be observed including musical components, facial expressions, movements, postures, reactivity (i.e., hyper, hypo), visual spatial capacities, motor-planning and sequencing abilities, and sensory sensitivities (e.g., tactile, vestibular, proprioception).

Each of the three scales that make up the IMCAP-ND are interconnected in that each examines different aspects of the client's capacities to musically interact. Therefore, in essence, each scale is attempting to dissect a musical interaction based on three interrelated categories— musical-emotional, cognition/perception, and preference, efficiency, and self-regulation— in order to provide an overall profile of the client's ability to relate and communicate in musical-play.

Thus, all aspects of each scale should be observed together while interacting with the client. For example, when observing and listening to a musical interaction the therapist should simultaneously be examining the client's musical-emotional capacity, cognitive and perceptual abilities, as well as the client's musical preferences, efficiency, and ability to self-regulate. The therapist should also be observing the client's media preferences and level of support being provided for particular target music responses.

When scoring the IMCAP-ND, all of its three scales may be scored individually or collectively. This is followed by an analysis of the data.

Therapist's Qualifications

The IMCAP-ND is designed for use by board-certified music therapists, as well as, music therapy students and interns under the guidance and/or supervision of a board-certified music therapist. Use of the IMCAP-ND is based on the therapist's clinical skills and understanding and experience with the assessment tool. Therapists administering the IMCAP-ND should be familiar with the ratings, fluent in clinical improvisation, and have a high level of clinical musicianship in order to focus their attention on clinical observation/listening. Therefore, music therapists must also be proficient in applying and understanding Bruscia's clinical techniques (Bruscia, 1987). (See Chapter 2.)

The relevance of the IMCAP-ND depends upon the clinical judgment of the therapist in regards to observational and listening skills as well as the decision making and implementation of musical and nonmusical interventions (i.e., level of support). In addition, therapists should have clinical experience with individuals with neurodevelopmental disorders.

Population-based

The IMCAP-ND is a population-specific assessment tool developed for working with children, adolescents, and adults with neurodevelopmental disorders to address core features of the disorder. The IMCAP-ND is designed to target and assess key aspects and features of neurodevelopmental disorders such as relating, communicating, emotionality, language, cognitive functioning, and sensory-motor processing.

Neurodevelopmental disorders include pervasive developmental disorders (PDD) also referred to as autism spectrum disorders; speech and language disorders and attention deficit-hyperactivity disorder (ADHD) (Tager-Flusberg & Helen, 1999). In addition, neurodevelopmental disorders include genetic disorders, such as fragile-X syndrome, Down's syndrome, Williams syndrome, Rett syndrome, and Angelman syndrome (ICDL, 2005; Tager-Flusberg & Helen, 1999; APA, 2000).

Core features of neurodevelopmental disorders generally impact communication, the ability to experience emotion (affect), language, cognitive functioning, sensory and motor processing, and in some cases impact relatedness (Zero to Three, 1994, 2005; Greenspan, 1992; ICDL, 2005; Tager-Flusberg & Helen, 1999).

Chapter 2: General Outline of Music Therapy Sessions

Summary of Chapter

Chapter 2 provides the therapist with a general outline of the music therapy sessions. The chapter begins by discussing the usual format for each session including length of session, how to approach the client musically and interpersonally, and media used by the therapist and client. In addition, musical-play and clinical improvisation are defined and discussed in terms of how the therapist applies and works in music to engage the client while also providing opportunities for interaction. Clinical techniques and procedural considerations are also presented, as well as three procedural phases that deal with the therapist–client musical process in musical-play. The chapter concludes by discussing intentionality in musical-play, how to work with perseverative behaviors, and procedures and categories of supportive interventions.

Session Format

Improvisational music therapy is provided in an individual setting, working one-to-one with the client. Generally, thirty to forty minutes are allotted for an assessment session; however, because each client responds and reacts differently to the new musical environment, the length of sessions may be shorter based on the client's ability to tolerate the new environment. Musical interactions are generally client-led and -directed, meaning that that musical experiences provided by the therapist are based on how the client is responding and reacting to those experiences. Hence, the therapist provides musical experiences based on the client's cues and emotions. However, based on the moment-to-moment interactions, or lack thereof, it may be indicated that the therapist introduce new musical ideas, guidance, and/or directions.

Musical Media

There are three forms of musical media explored when administering the IMCAP-ND: 1) instrument, 2) vocal, and 3) movement. During the assessment the client has a wide range of musical instruments available including drums, conga, cymbals, xylophone, xylimba, reed horns, tambourines, floor tom, and various other percussive instruments. The client may vocalize or sing. In addition, the client's spontaneous movement responses are continuously observed and incorporated into the therapist's music. Clients are generally given free choice of musical media and instruments at all times.

The therapist may use any combination of drums, tambourine, cymbal, or other pitched or unpitched percussive instrument as well as voice, guitar, or piano. Instruments are selected by the therapist based on the client's moment-to-moment musical responses.

Musical-Play

Musical-play is at the heart of the IMCAP-ND. It provides clients with creative and relational opportunities that are indigenous to music making while generating here-and-now musical events. Thus, it is in musical-play that the therapist is observing and listening to the client's ability to perceive, comprehend, respond, interact, and self-regulate.

The IMCAP-ND defines musical-play as a form of interaction that involves two or more participants engaged in coactive music making. It may include any one or a combination of four types of music experiences (methods) including improvising, re-creating, composing, and (active) listening (Bruscia, 1998). For the purpose of administering the IMCAP-ND, however, improvisational music experiences will be the main music therapy method discussed in this manual. The IMCAP-ND identifies three media of musical expression in musical-play: 1) instruments, 2) vocalizing, and 3) movement. Thus, the therapist and client may interact in musical-play through any one or a combination of the three media.

Chapter 2: General Outline of Music Therapy Sessions

The clinical application of musical-play requires the therapist to musically approach each client in a manner that is respectful of their neurological and musical differences. Therefore, therapists are required to be musically flexible in their ability to offer clients a variety of musical contexts through a wide range of musical elements (e.g., tempo, dynamics, harmony, melody, etc.) in order to provide clients with many opportunities to display their strengths and areas of difficulty.

To summarize, in order to assess cognitive and interactive musical processes, the therapist must be able to move freely within various musical dimensions while differentiating musical elements (e.g., tempo, dynamics, etc.) and at the same time responding to the client with true spontaneous empathy rather than stock musical responses.

Clinical Improvisation

Musical-play involving spontaneous back-and-forth musical dialoguing between the client and therapist may be best facilitated through the use of clinical improvisation (Nordoff & Robbins, 2007; Bruscia, 1987). In the improvisational approaches (Alvin & Warwick, 1991; Nordoff & Robbins, 2007; Wigram, 2004; Bryan, 1989; Saperston, 1973; Wimpory, Chadwick, & Nash, 1995), therapists usually employ a nondirective approach using clinical improvisation on a variety of instruments, and movement with music to address areas involving self-expression, communication, body awareness, anxiety and aggression, sensory integration, socialization, and communication.

In clinical improvisation, the therapist follows the client's musical lead and extemporaneously creates music to further engage the client's musical and nonmusical responses. Put another way, the therapist places every response the client offers, either intentionally or reflexively, within a musical framework, which then enables them to interact and develop their own unique therapist–client relationship. By doing so, the therapist gains insight into the client's musical-emotional strengths and challenges. In addition, through these improvisation experiences, the client may reveal individual skill differences that impede engaging in higher levels of musical-play, which then gives the therapist information needed to design and employ the most effective supportive interventions.

Clinical Techniques

A key feature of the IMCAP-ND deals with understanding the client's musical responses in the context of relating and communicating during improvisatory sessions. Thus, music therapists administering the IMCAP-ND must be proficient at responding musically while implementing clinical techniques.

Bruscia (1987) identifies sixty-four clinical techniques used in improvisational music therapy that are grouped into nine specific categories: 1) techniques of empathy, 2) structuring techniques, 3) techniques of intimacy, 4) elicitation techniques, 5) redirection techniques, 6) procedural techniques, 7) emotional exploratory techniques, 8) referential techniques, and 9) discussion techniques. Due to the nature of the IMCAP-ND and the client group that it is intended for, this manual will focus only on techniques of empathy, structuring techniques, techniques of intimacy, elicitation techniques, and redirection techniques. Clinical techniques used by the therapist vary according to which target music response is being examined as well as the moment-to-moment interactions.

Empathy techniques involve the therapist imitating, pacing, reflecting, and/or synchronizing with what the client is doing while capturing the mood, feeling, and emotion that he/she may be expressing. Exaggerating and incorporating are also techniques of empathy in which the therapist musically uses and/or brings out the client's musical motif or a distinct musical response.

When implementing structuring techniques, the therapist may provide rhythmic grounding (foundation), tonal centering, and/or shaping in which the therapist enhances the client's music.

Techniques of intimacy include the therapist sharing the same instrument with the client (share instruments), and/or providing him/her with a musical gift, i.e., performance (giving). The therapist may also create a clinical theme that is based on the therapeutic relationship (bonding) and/or improvise a song about the client (soliloquies).

Elicitation techniques are comprised of the therapist repeating, extending, and/or completing a musical idea or component that is presented by the client. They may also include the therapist modeling something for the client to imitate, and/or interjecting a musical idea, and/or leaving space in the music for the client to respond.

Redirection techniques involve the therapist imposing musical changes (e.g., rhythms, meter, melodies, tonality, lyrics, etc.) within a musical experience and/or playing music that is distinctly different from the client's music yet related (differentiating). Offering an increase or decrease in tempo, dynamics, and/or harmonic and melodic tension are also used to redirect and focus the client to a musical task.

Procedural Considerations

The following procedures and considerations should be applied by the therapist throughout the assessment process when administering the IMCAP-ND:

- Determine what instrument to play, or whether to sing based on the moment-to-moment interactions while considering a particular target music response that needs to be assessed.

- Determine if "enough" musical opportunities have been provided for the client in order to accurately assess a particular target music response.

- Determine if musical experiences have included a variety and a range of musical elements, contexts, and arrangements.

- Determine if musical contexts and arrangement of musical experiences are client centered or client driven.

- Determine if the client requires support (i.e., verbal, visual, and/or physical) in order to demonstrate capacity in a particular target music response.

- Determine if the client requires particular sensory support or input (e.g., tactile, proprioceptive, and or/vestibular, etc.) in musical-play in order to demonstrate capacity in a particular target music response.

- Ensure that if support is required that it is provided from least to most (i.e., verbal is considered least while physical is most).

- Determine the rate of frequency of a client's response in a particular target music area.

- Determine the media in which the client offered a target music response.

Procedural Phases

The course of improvising musical experiences throughout the IMCAP-ND process involves three phases: 1) following client's lead, 2) two-way purposeful musical-play, and 3) affect synchrony in musical-play. Informed by the Developmental, Individual-Differences, Relationship-based (DIR®)/ Floortime™ Model (Greenspan, 1992) and Nordoff-Robbins Music Therapy (NRMT) (Nordoff & Robbins, 2007), these progressive work phases provide the therapist with a guide to musically approach and analyze clients in terms of target music responses. Each phase is identified by its own objectives and techniques and each requires different developmental skills on the part of the client. Therefore, the client's developmental capacity for musical-play will determine the working phase or phases of the session.

As shown in Figure 4, the therapist follows and moves through a sequence of stages to achieve each phase, always beginning and reverting back to the first phase, following the client's musical-emotional lead.

Figure 4. Procedural Phases

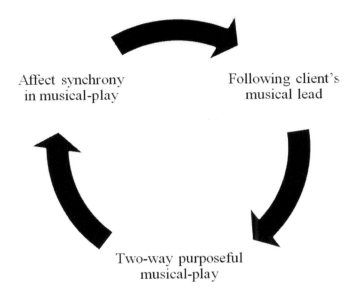

Following the client's musical emotional lead

Following the client's lead is a Floortime™ technique (Greenspan, 1992; Greenspan & Weider, 2006a, 2006b) that refers to the therapist following the client's natural emotional interests while at the same time challenging him/her socially, emotionally, and intellectually. Greenspan (1992) explains that by focusing on the client's interests while following his/her lead, the therapist is invited into the client's emotional life (1992). Thus, by following a client's natural desires, the therapist can begin to understand what the client finds enjoyable and pleasurable (Greenspan & Weider, 2006a, 2006b). Musically, this is no different. By following the client's musical emotional lead, the therapist can begin to understand the client musically in terms of his/her musical tendencies, preferred choice of musical media, and the overall types of musical experiences (e.g., styles, idioms, contexts, etc.) that he/she finds pleasurable.

Nordoff and Robbins (2007) referred to the same phase in their work with children with special needs. They called the phase "meeting the client musically," in which musical engagement begins with matching the client's emotional "being" or state with the music. Thus, the therapist improvises music that accepts and meets the client, musically, and in doing so opens a channel of communication (Aigen, 2005; Nordoff & Robbins, 2007).

The aims of this phase are to build rapport with the client by creating an accepting musical environment that is respectful of his/her reactions and responses; this will help the therapist to discover the client's musical tendencies, preferences, sensitivities, and preferred musical media and discern what the client finds pleasurable and unpleasant in musical-play.

Following the client's musical-emotional lead begins by observing and listening to his/her reactions, responses, and initiated behaviors. During this phase the therapist is seeking out clues and cues that will inform the musical direction of the interaction. Thus, the therapist is watching and listening to how the client: a) separates from his/her parents or caregiver, b) enters into the room, and c) is experiencing the musical environment and situation. Prior to the therapist playing and/or singing a note, he/she may begin to conceptualize the client musically and begin planning a framework for a musical experience based on observable and/or audible responses and reactions. The therapist may initially focus on the client's awareness of tempo, rhythm, and pace of motor movements (e.g., walking, pacing, running, jumping, utilization of the instruments, etc.) while being attentive to any vocal sounds being expressed (reflexive and/or intentional). In addition, the therapist at the same time is observing which instrument the client is drawn to and the manner in which client approaches, handles, and/or plays the instrument.

In this work phase the therapist is being attentive to the client's emotional climate as well as his/her ability to process the sensory information in the environment while seeking to answer questions such as:

- Is the client self-directed?

- Does the client maneuver with a look of fear and/or ambivalence?

- How does the client physically (motor) and perceptually maneuver around the room?

- Does the client present with no fear?

- Does the client display awareness to physical and interpersonal boundaries?

- Does the client move repeatedly from one instrument to the next?

- Does the client display an interest in any of the instruments, music, and/or therapist?

- Is the client's interest in the instruments motivated by sensory or musical desires?

- Does the client handle and play the instruments with their intended purpose?

- What is the client's overall reactivity level (i.e., hypo, hyper, or mixed) during the musical experience?

- Is the client approachable musically and/or interpersonally?

- What are the client's musical tendencies and preferences in terms of musical style, idioms, elements, form, and context?

Musically, the therapist follows the client's lead (based on clinical observation and listening) by improvising music that meets or matches the client's affect while accompanying, reflecting, synchronizing, and/or enhancing any musical and nonmusical responses and reactions that the client may be expressing. All client responses and reactions, including idiosyncratic perseverative behaviors, are viewed and heard as communicative and are conceptualized within a musical context. Thus, the therapist musically responds to the client's moment-to-moment responses or behaviors, while consistently matching his/her affect as means of acceptance.

Meeting perseverative behaviors

Many clients with neurodevelopmental challenges repeat themselves and engage in perseverative behavior patterns. These repetitive patterns can manifest musically (e.g., perseverative beating on a percussive instrument, echolalia, repeatedly vocalizing song lyrics that are out of context, etc.) and/or physically (e.g., hand flapping, pacing, etc.). In all of its forms, the therapist's task is to accept and perceive these behavior patterns as communicative and to musically join the client. This may include the therapist improvising music within the tempo of the client's hand flapping, or creating a musical form built around a perseverative vocalization. It may also include the therapist singing improvised song lyrics that are related to the client's repetitive verbalizations.

The music in this phase should be unintrusive, unimposing, and flexible in order for it to maintain consistency with the client's affect while allowing the client to lead the interaction. Thus, tempo and dynamics are generally stable while rhythms are kept simple and related to the beat. Harmonic frameworks are tonally centered and include clear cadences. Melody is created with the intent to create a theme or motif. Melodic themes and motifs are introduced in a clear manner and are generally repeated. Themes may be repeated in their original form and/or through a variation. The use of voice is introduced based on the clinical judgment of the moment-to-moment situation; the choice to incorporate lyrics and/or nonverbal singing is dependent upon the client's capacity to process verbal information as well as informed by the implication of the clinical situation.

Clinical techniques used to follow the client's emotional lead may be any one or a combination of the empathy and/or structuring techniques (Bruscia, 1987). These techniques of empathy include imitating, synchronizing, incorporating, pacing, reflecting, and exaggerating. Structuring techniques include rhythmic grounding, tonal centering, and shaping. The empathy and structuring techniques are incorporated into the improvisation to match and reflect the client's affect and actions (musical and nonmusical), facial and body expressions, and movements to music.

Two-way purposeful music making

In the second phase, the therapist works to create music experiences that provide opportunities for the client to engage in two-way purposeful communication (Greenspan & Weider, 2006a, 2006b). This involves the therapist musically opening circles of communication (Greenspan, 1992) for the client to respond. Circles of communication are called "circles" because they involve give-and-take interactions in which both communicators are reciprocating to one another (Greenspan & Weider, 2006a, 2006b) within a particular context. Therefore, in order for there to be communication, the receiver of the dialogue needs to respond back to the initiator of the circle.

The therapist working in this phase is paying close attention to the quality of musical interactions in order to determine:

- Is there a continuous flow (Greenspan, 1992; Greenspan & Weider, 2006a, 2006b) to the musical-play?

- Do the musical interactions contain mutuality in tempo, rhythm, and affect?

- Can the client open and/or close circles of musical communication via any musical media? (A circle of musical communication involve reciprocity in which both therapist and client are responding to one another in a mutual and intentional manner.)

- Does the client display an understanding of cause-and-effect relationship in musical-play?

- Does the client exhibit the ability to differentiate between his/her own music and the therapist's?

Musically, when working in this phase, the therapist improvises based on the client's lead, then offers or expresses a musical question, statement, and/or partial statement seeking a musical response. Therefore, in this phase the therapist initiates a musical offering whereby he/she is now leading or guiding the interaction.

The critical feature of working in this phase is knowing when and how to transition from the first phase into phase two. Criteria for moving into phase two involves the therapist's understanding of the observable and audible relational dynamics occurring within the musical interaction in regards to the client's intent, desire, musical tendencies, and emotional stability and range. Therefore, prior to this transition the client should be exhibiting self-regulation, shared attention and shared affect, and engagement within the musical interaction. At any time during or after the transition into phase two, the therapist may revert back to phase one if the client exhibits difficulty transitioning and/or withdraws from the interaction. In that case the therapist may return to following the client's lead while formulating an alternative musical strategy before attempting to transition into phase two.

Creating a musical opportunity for two-way purposeful communication always begins with following the client's lead and meeting him/her musically. This is followed by the therapist making the transition into phase two by creating a musical offering, i.e., a musical question, or a partial or completed musical statement (opening a circle of communication) that is consistent with the original musical idea, while at the same time seeking a response (closing circle of communication) from the client.

The musical characteristics when working in this phase should be moderately intrusive and imposing to some degree, in order for the therapist to create a musical offering to the client. It is also important that the music be flexible and capable of changing direction. Tempo and dynamics should be flexible and mobile, while rhythms are either kept simple and related to the beat, or may include syncopation and other complex forms. Harmonic frameworks can be tonally or atonally centered and may or may not include clear cadences. In addition, tonality and harmony should be flexible and capable of modulating. Melodic themes and motifs may be used in their original or varied form. The voice may be expressed using a wide range of affect and timbre based on the clinical situation. As in phase one, the choice to incorporate lyrics and/or nonverbal singing is dependent upon the client's capacity to process verbal information as well as being informed by the clinical situation. Overall, when working in this phase, the music should be flexible, mobile, and capable of being multidimensional while at the same time provide the client with an offering.

Clinical techniques utilized in this phase may include any combination of empathy and structuring techniques while incorporating elicitation and redirection techniques (Bruscia, 1987).

Elicitation techniques include repeating, modeling, making spaces, interjecting, extending, and completing. Redirection techniques include introducing change, differentiating, modulating, intensifying, calming, intervening, imitating, synchronizing, incorporating, pacing, reflecting, and exaggerating. Structuring techniques include rhythmic grounding, tonal centering, and shaping.

The overall purpose of the indicated techniques is to elicit some sort of response that is related to the music being offered by the therapist. The response may manifest through a glance, tap on the drum or cymbal (or other instrument), groan, movement, facial expression, or of course through conventional music making. The key feature is that the response is intentional and related to the music.

Affect synchrony in musical-play

As the client engages in related musical experiences, he/she begins to recognize and respond to musical cues such as changes in tempo, dynamics, phrasing, timbre, as well as music-based movement (e.g., motion, gestures, etc.). Through these musically mutual experiences the client and therapist begin to engage in two-way purposeful musical-play; the client demonstrates intentionality in his/her music making that is directly related to the therapist's music. Once this occurs, the therapist may now begin planning to transition into phase three, affect synchrony (Feldman, 2007), which is described as the matching of affective behavior between parent and child as both engage in a "continuous dance" (p. 602) to maintain a patterned relationship throughout play.

In the context of therapist–client, the affect synchrony musical-play phase involves the client initiating and responding to musical ideas and cues via a range of musical media while engaging in long chains of back-and-forth reciprocal affective interactions (Greenspan & Shanker, 2004).

It has been theorized that individuals with neurodevelopmental disorders, specifically autism, lack the developmental capacity to connect affect (emotion or intent) to motor planning and sequencing, thus making it difficult to engage in sustained reciprocal affective interactions (Greenspan & Shanker, 2004; Greenspan, 1992; Greenspan & Weider, 2006b; Feldman, 2007).

This phase deals with the therapist creating musical experiences that will provide the client with the opportunities to demonstrate the capacity to initiate, respond, and engage in a continuous flow of robust and affective musical interactions.

Generally, when working in this phase, the therapist is focusing on three specific areas: 1) quality of musical-play interactions, 2) intent of actions in musical-play, and 3) range of musical-play.

Quality of musical-play interactions

Observing the quality of musical-play interactions in phase three involves the therapist determining the client's intent, tendencies, and general patterns of interactions based on four categories: 1) fragmented and intermittent (no consistent pattern), 2) fragmented and cyclical (consistent pattern), 3) continuous but constricted in tempo and dynamic range, and 4) continuous through a range of tempo and dynamics.

Fragmented and intermittent (no consistent pattern)

When a client musically interacts in a fragmented and intermittent manner with no consistent pattern, he/she will engage in two-way purposeful musical-play and display some capacity to musically engage, although, the musical-play lacks a continuous flow of reciprocal interactions. Thus, interactions may consist of fleeting moments of related musical interactions in which the client may engage briefly. This is followed by the client withdrawing from the interaction via self-stimulatory behaviors, and/or physically moving away from the interaction, and/or emotionally withdrawing (e.g., crying, anxious laughing, screaming, etc.), and/or sensory processing challenges (hyper- or hyporesponsive). In addition, clients engaging in an intermittent and fragmented manner with no consistent pattern may not rejoin the interaction unless supported by the therapist.

Fragmented and cyclical (consistent pattern)

When a client musically interacts in a fragmented and cyclical manner within a consistent pattern, he/she will interact in two-way purposeful musical-play and demonstrate capacity to musically engage, although, here too, the musical-play lacks a continuous flow of reciprocal interactions. Clients engaging in this category will withdraw from interactions, but will typically return to the interaction and rejoin musical-play with the therapist.

Continuous but constricted in tempo and dynamic range

When a client is able to musically engage in a continuous manner but is constricted in tempo and dynamic range, he/she may display the ability to musically relate for a sustained period, although, the range of play exhibits limitations in tempo and dynamics. Thus, when the client is presented with musical experiences that include a range of tempo and dynamics, he/she may withdraw physically (moving away), and/or musically (e.g., maintaining the original tempo/dynamic and/or the change overloads the client's sensory system in which he/she becomes disorganized and dysregulated), and/or emotionally (e.g., becoming angry, sad, excited, anxious, etc.).

Continuous through a range of tempo and dynamics

When a client is able to musically engage in musical-play in a continuous manner through a range of tempo and dynamics, the interactions are robust and flowing, with a clear give-and-take between the therapist and client. Clients may display this capacity in one and/or two ways: 1) when the therapist introduces (initiates) musical changes that include a range in tempo and dynamics and/or 2) when the client introduces (initiates) musical changes pertaining to tempo and dynamics.

Range in musical-play

A critical feature of musical interaction that needs to be closely evaluated is range. Range refers to the client's capacity to engage in related music making that includes a variety of tempo, dynamics, and other expressive musical elements. Therefore, a client may demonstrate the ability to musically relate in a continuous flowing manner for extended periods when the music is played in a fast tempo (allegro), but may display difficulty sustaining musical relatedness at a slower tempo. Furthermore, some clients may demonstrate the ability to engage in mutual music making only when the musical experience incorporates staccato playing and/or singing, or may only display the ability to engage when the music is fast or slow. These examples portray clients who although they have the capacity to musically engage in a robust and continuous manner, have a limited range and a limited or one-dimensional ability to engage in mutual music making.

Intentionality in musical-play

In assessing intentionality, one may argue that all responses are intentional in some form. Defining specifically what is heard and/or observed as being intentional is very important when scoring the IMCAP-ND. For example, a client may walk into the therapy room and begin beating a drum while being completely oblivious of the therapist's presence. His/her intent was to beat the drum. Therefore, the therapist may view this as a display of intentional playing. The IMCAP-ND, however, views intentionality within the context of relating and communicating to another person and their music. Therefore, intentionality is being assessed based on the client's ability to engage in musical-play with the intent to relate and/or communicate musically and interpersonally with the therapist.

For example, a client walks into the therapy room and begins playing a reed horn as he turns and glances toward the therapist. The therapist picks up on the musical and interpersonal cues and begins to create music to accompany the horn and foster musical mutuality, relatedness, and communication. Both therapist and client are engaged in a mutual musical experience. The client continues to blow the reed horn while watching the therapist and increasing the dynamic of his horn playing. The therapist follows the client's musical lead by increasing the dynamic while initiating an increase in tempo. The client begins to play faster, adapting his playing to the therapist's music. Finally, the therapist gradually decreases the tempo. The client follows the decrease of tempo and the musical experience comes to an end. Immediately following the conclusion of the musical experience, the client socially references the therapist with a glance and a smile.

Musically, when working in this phase (affect synchrony), it is recommended that the music be supportive and flexible in order for the therapist to be able to shift and change the music depending on the clinical situation at hand. Dynamics and tempo should be kept constant and based on the client's responses and preferences. Rhythms should be kept simple and anchored to the basic beat, but also be flexible in case the therapist or client choose to relinquish the pulse of the music. Harmonically the music should be tonally centered; chords should be indicative to the direction of the harmony and melody with repetition used throughout to create predictability and form. Changes in the music should be subtle and variations of the repeated themes should be incorporated.

The voice should be used throughout while being the main vehicle for melody, range of timbre, and affect. The implementation of lyrics and/or nonverbal singing is based on the client's developmental level and clinical situation. Although harmonic accompaniment should include the guitar or piano, percussive instruments may be used, if indicated, to support the therapist's singing. In all of its forms, these musical components are kept consistent with the client's emotional being and clinical situation.

Clinical techniques utilized in this phase include a range of empathy, structuring, elicitation, redirection, and intimacy (Bruscia, 1987). (See phase one and two for techniques of empathy, structuring, and redirection.) Intimacy techniques include sharing instruments, giving, bonding, and soliloquies.

Procedures for Supportive Interventions

Individuals with neurodevelopmental disorders generally display difficulty learning from everyday experiences. Therefore, they may experience challenges when responding to musical and interpersonal cues in musical-play.

Therapists should observe and listen for cues in musical-play in order to determine the type of support and the intensity in which it will be delivered in order for the client to demonstrate a particular target music response. The task of the therapist when administering supportive interventions is to help the client exhibit a response while providing feedback and a variety of musical opportunities for the client to display the particular target music response.

Although rating and scoring supportive intervention levels are specific to Scale I: Musical Emotional Assessment Rating Scale (MEARS), they may be implemented throughout the entire session and therefore must be applied in a sequential manner. The author has identified a hierarchy of three categories of supportive interventions beginning with the least to most support. They include: 1) verbal, 2) visual, and 3) physical (Cooper, Heron, & Heward, 2007). The hierarchy of supportive interventions provides a systematic method of assisting clients as well as provide a framework to understanding their level of independence while engaged in musical-play.

As mentioned above, supportive interventions should be provided in the order of least to most support and should only be implemented after the therapist has provided the client with many musical contexts and experiences that allow for opportunities to display a particular target music response.

When it is indicated that the client requires support, the therapist will begin the intervention by offering verbal cuing (minimal support) within musical-play. This may include incorporating words into the music experience that ask the client to do something, and/or reflect what the client is doing, and/or repeat or echo what the client is saying or singing. If the client still appears to have difficulty attending to verbal cues, the next level (mild) of support, visual cuing, should be embedded into musical-play.

Embedding visual support within musical-play includes the therapist cuing the client through gesture, and/or pointing, and/or affective facial expressions and/or body movements, and/or positioning an instrument in front of the client. If the client continues to display difficulty providing the target music response, the therapist will then provide partial physical support (moderate) in musical-play. This involves the therapist physically guiding the client gently and sensitively to a particular area of the room or an instrument. It may also involve the therapist gently nudging the client at the time of the desired target music response. Finally, if the client continues to exhibit difficulty in displaying a target music response, full physical assistance (maximum support) may be indicated. This involves providing the client with a hand-over-hand (HOH) technique while he/she is playing an instrument, such as holding the client's hand and gently and playfully bringing him/her to a particular place in the room and/or by guiding their hand in musical-play in order to experience the target music response.

Minimal support

"Minimal support" includes verbal cues and/or directions. This may include the therapist incorporating verbal cuing into the musical-play as a means to foster interaction while assessing the client's needs and strengths in musical-play.

Verbal cues

During musical-play, verbal cues can be incorporated in lyrical or spoken form in order to guide and/or redirect the client during musical interactions, such as:

- Vocally (verbally) guide the client in musical-play regarding changes in tempo, dynamics, melody, etc.

- Vocally (verbally) redirecting a client who may be displaying difficulty maintaining focus in musical-play.

- Vocally (verbally) demonstrate the desired musical response.

- Vocally (verbally) demonstrate only a part of the musical response.

Mild support

"Mild support" consists of visual cues that include physical modeling, gestures, and/or positional (Cooper, Heron, & Heward, 2007) supportive interventions.

Modeling

Clients who display the ability to learn and engage in imitation may benefit from the therapist modeling a desired response on a particular instrument, and/or nonverbal vocalizing, and/or via movement. Modeling can be incorporated in musical-play and employed by the therapist by:

- Demonstrating how to play or hold a particular instrument, and/or vocalize (nonverbally) a particular melodic line, and/or make a specific movement to the music.

- Demonstrating within the interaction while engaged in music making, the therapist may model when to play, sing, and/or move whereby eliciting a specific musical response (e.g., punctuating the end or beginning of a musical phrase).

- Demonstrating a rhythmic pattern within the interaction for the client to repeat.

Gesture

In providing affect/gesture as a supportive strategy in musical-play, the therapist is essentially utilizing a physical or emotional (affective) cue to help the client musically respond to a specific musical experience. Thus, the therapist is paying close attention to the moment-to-moment interactions regarding the client's ability to musically respond in an intentional and affective manner. Clients that require high affect in order to engage in musical-play may present as being lethargic, passive, and inactively unresponsive to the music being presented. In addition, clients who respond musically in a reflexive manner and display a flat affect may benefit from musical experiences and gestures that include high affect.

Musical experiences that are charged with high affect may be used in tandem with over exaggerated body movements, gestures, and/or facial expressions in order to foster musical engagement and interaction. To embed high affect in musical-play, the therapist may incorporate a wide range of musical elements and/or singing styles, including:

- Glissandos.
- Chord clusters.
- Dissonance in chord structures.
- A wide range of tempo and dynamic changes.
- Detached and unpredictable playing.
- Singing in a jovial manner.
- Variations of strumming patterns and/or attack.

- A wide range of vocal sounds, including variation of timbre, while singing.

- Musical expereinces that contain forms and/or structures that are unpredictable.

Some clients may be more musically responsive and engaged when the therapist offers gestural cues during musical-play. Incorporating gestures in musical-play can emotionally "charge" the musical interaction by over/or under exaggerating a particular moment in the musical experience. Gestural cues incorporated into musical-play may include:

- Using over/or under exaggerated hand and/or arm movements in the general direction of the client and/or while playing an instrument in musical-play in order to indicate musical changes and/or to cue the client.

- Utilizing a range of facial expressions that convey a range of emotions (e.g., sad, excited, overjoyed, etc.) in order to foster musical engagement, and/or indicate musical changes (e.g., dynamics, tempo, etc.), and/or cue the client.

Positional

Generally, most interactions in musical-play involve instruments. To utilize a positional supportive intervention (Cooper, Heron, & Heward, 2007), the therapist can move the instrument closer to the client at the time of the target music response in musical-play. Thus, the therapist is positioning the instrument or object within the client's physical and visual range. (Hand slapping in musical-play can also be utilized when offering positional support.)

Moderate support

"Moderate support" consists of partial physical assistance (Cooper, Heron, & Heward, 2007) being implemented to foster musical-play.

Partial physical support

When engaging a client in musical-play, the therapist partially assists the client by guiding his/her hand to an instrument in order to foster a specific musical response. This may also include guiding the client's elbow in the form of a gentle nudge to help him/her to execute a specific musical response.

Maximum support

"Maximum support" consists of full physical assistance or hand-over-hand (HOH) (Cooper, Heron, & Heward, 2007) being implemented to foster musical-play.

Full physical support

When working with a client who presents as being underreactive, passive, timid, and/or insecure the hand-over-hand (HOH) technique can help guide them into a musical experience that otherwise they may be unable to engage in independently. Clients who display with perceptual challenges, motor difficulties, and/or visual impairments can benefit from HOH support (Nordoff & Robbins, 2007). Providing HOH support can help a client physically go through the motions of playing an instrument while providing them with the feel, action, and experience of making music. When providing HOH support it is important that the therapist be extremely sensitive to the degree of physical effort that the client is putting into this joint effort (Nordoff & Robbins, 2007).

HOH support can be provided in several forms. For example, the therapist may provide HOH in musical-play by holding and guiding the client's hands, and/or gently holding and directing the client's forearm and wrist, and/or holding and guiding the client's bicep/s (Nordoff & Robbins, 2007).

While providing hand-over-hand support during the musical interaction, the therapist should be mindful of:

- The physical effort that the client is putting toward playing.

- When to provide more or less effort while offering this support.

- The client's comfort level in regards to being touched.

- The client's motivation (e.g., is it increasing or decreasing?).

- How to guide the client's playing by:

    - Supporting him/her in beating the basic beat.

    - Supporting him/her in punctuating the beginning and/or end of a musical phrase.

    - Supporting him/her in experiencing tempo and/or dynamic changes.

    - Supporting him/her in experiencing a meter change.

    - Supporting him/her in experiencing a particular accent and/or articulation.

    - Supporting him/her in experiencing a particular melody on the piano, xylophone, and/or other particular instrument.

    - Supporting him/her in experiencing a particular strum pattern on the guitar.

Chapter 3
Scale I: Musical Emotional Assessment Rating Scale

Summary of Chapter

This chapter introduces the therapist to the Musical Emotional Assessment Rating Scale (MEARS). It includes a detailed description of the MEARS, criteria for target responses, protocols and procedures, clinical techniques, considerations, and scoring instructions. The MEARS examines the client's ability to musically attend, respond affectively, adapt, engage, and interrelate (see Figure 5). Scoring is based on frequency of response, support provided for response, and media in which the client offered the response.

Figure 5. Example of the MEARS evaluating the client's ability to adapt in musical-play

III. ADAPTION TO MUSICAL-PLAY	Frequency	Support	Media
e) Joins	4	5	I,V
f) Adjusts	4	3	I,V
g) Takes Turns	2	3	I
h) Stops	2	4	I,M
Totals/Avg.	12/3	15/3.75	I,V,M

Musical Emotional Assessment Rating Scale (MEARS)

The Musical Emotional Assessment Rating Scale (MEARS) is a criterion-referenced instrument designed to assess and evaluate the client's musical-emotional responsiveness in musical-play based on five music domain areas: 1) *musical attention*, 2) *musical affect*, 3) *adaption to musical-play*, 4) *musical engagement*, and 5) *musical interrelatedness*. The developmental sequence of the five areas is informed by Greenspan's Functional Emotional Developmental Levels (Greenspan, DeGangi, & Weider, 2001), the DIR®/Floortime™ Model, as well as the author's task analysis of the relative difficulty of each musical capacity (Carpente, 2009, 2011, 2012). Although each area is relevant to neurodevelopmental disorders, the sequence of musical capacities (domain areas) may or may not be consistent with musical development in typical developing children.

Level I: Musical Attention

The beginning of any interaction starts with being attentive for engagement and interaction. The ability to engage in meaningful and intentional music making requires the capacity to be emotionally and cognitively available and prepared to interact. Being musically available involves maintaining readiness, alertness, and availability to engage while at the same time processing the musical experience. Furthermore, it includes the capacity to maintain calmness while controlling impulses through a wide range of musical and sensory experiences (e.g., auditory, visual, proprioception, tactile, etc.). Musical attention deals with understanding how the client attends to musical-play based on four categories:

- Focuses: how the client attends to one or more aspects of therapist, music, or play.

- Maintains: how the client sustains attention to one particular aspect of therapist, music, or play.

- Shares: how the client sustains attention to one particular aspect of therapist, music, or play also being attended by therapist.

- Shifts: how the client changes attentional focus to match the attentional focus of the therapist.

Assessing Musical Attention

Instructions

Begin to assess capacities for musical attention by attempting to engage the client musically, always following his/her emotional lead. While creating musical experiences for the client, pay attention to visible and audible cues, such as the tempo and rhythm of his/her movement, facial expressions, vocalizations, emotional climate, and the focus of his/her attention. Shift the musical experiences based on the client's responses and behaviors so that the music is matching the general mood of the client as well as his/her responses and behaviors. When improvising around the client's responses it is recommended that you create a clear musical form (e.g., A-B-A, etc.). This may be followed by repeating one or more of the musical components (e.g., melody, melodic rhythm, motif, etc.) within the original framework in order to create predictability.

Introduce your voice within the musical framework. The style and timbre of your voice should be compatible with the musical framework as well as related to the client's responses and behaviors. Depending on the client's developmental level and clinical situation, it is suggested that you incorporate words/lyrics into the improvisation that include the client's name, and/or reflect what the client is doing, and/or as a means to direct the client's attention (e.g., verbal support). During the musical experience it is important to pay close attention to the client's reactions and responses to determine if he/she is processing and taking in the sights and sounds of the musical environment. In addition, it is imperative to alter the music if the client is becoming dysregulated (hyper- or hyporeactive) by the musical experience being presented. You may need to shift the musical experience, including media, accordingly.

Other strategies to evoke musical attention include incorporating contrasting music that is related to an original theme and form. In addition, offering the client a different instrument, or adding a second or third instrument into the musical-play, may be a way of facilitating attention (shift). In all of its forms, the musical strategies employed are based on the client's emotional lead and are focused on providing musical opportunities for the client to display the ability to musically attend.

If the client does not exhibit the target response after being provided with multiple musical contexts through a range of musical components, it is suggested that supportive interventions be embedded into the musical experience (i.e., verbal, visual, and physical). (See Chapter 2 regarding procedures for providing supportive interventions.)

Clinical techniques

Assessing musical attention involves the implementation of clinical techniques that are focused on following the client's lead, creating a musical framework, and evoking musical responses. Therefore, it is recommended that the following clinical techniques be used: imitating, synchronizing, incorporating, pacing, reflecting, exaggerating, rhythmic grounding, tonal centering, sharing instruments, repeating, making spaces, extending, and/or completing (Bruscia, 1987).

Considerations

In addition to observing target responses, the therapist should be considering the client's preferences and individual differences that may be interfering with his/her ability to musically attend. The following questions should be considered during clinical observations/listening:

- What is the client's preferred and least preferred musical context or arrangement in musical-play in regards to musical attention?

- What is the client's preferred and least preferred type of support (verbal, visual, and/or physical) in musical-play in regards to musical attention?

- Does the client display an interest in the instruments in regards to musical attention?

    - What instrument/s is the client most and least interested in?

    - Does the client exhibit difficulty attending while holding mallets in musical-play?

    - Can the client play his/her preferred instrument while maintaining musical attention?

- Can the client display musical attention for a consistent period of time while musically engaged? When not musically engaged?

- Does the client display poor gait and balance, and if so, how is this impacting his/her ability to musically attend?

- Does the client display poor muscle tone, and if so, how is this impacting his/her ability to musically attend?

- Does the client display poor motor-planning and sequencing skills, and if so, how is this impacting his/her ability to musically attend?

- What is the client's reactivity level (i.e., hypo, hyper, and/or mixed) during musical-play and how does it impact his/her ability to attend?

- Is the client in constant motion (craving movement) in musical-play, and if so, how is this impacting his/her ability to musically attend?
  - Walking back and forth in a line?
  - Walking in circular motion?
  - Jumping up and down?
  - Does the client bump into things?

Level II: Musical Affect

Human emotion (affect) is consistently implicated in the practice of music therapy (Aigen, 2005). Expressing or experiencing affect (emotion) in musical-play provides various kinds of meaning to the musical task at hand. If the client is only engaged in musical-play on a sensory-motor level, he/she may exhibit difficulty in experiencing and integrating the relational, expressive, and communicative components of musical-play. Clients that can experience musical-play on an affective level may begin to show capacity in the ability to initiate, form ideas, and seek out relationships. Musical affect deals with how the client responds affectively in musical-play regarding four areas:

- Facial: expresses affect facially in response to therapist, music, or play.

- Prosody: expresses affect with voice in response to therapist, music, or play.

- Body: expresses affect through stationary movement in response to therapist, music, or play.

- Motion: expresses affect by moving toward or away from something in response to therapist, music, or play.

Assessing Musical Affect

Instructions

Once the client displays focused attention in musical-play, continue to musically follow his/her interests. Maintain musical consistency and predictability to ensure that the client feels comfortable and accepted. As the shared musical experience extends, pay attention to the client's overall affect. If there are variations and changes in the client's affect during musical-play, begin shifting the music in order to meet the client's affect while noticing if the affect is congruent with the musical experience. If the client engages musically while exhibiting flat or fixed affect, begin to alter the music by manipulating musical components until any form of affect is being expressed. This may involve increasing or decreasing tempo, changing the rhythm, modulating tonality, and creating contrasting music. Other musical changes to evoke affective responses may include exaggerating various musical components (within the context of the original musical framework), introducing syncopated rhythms and anticipatory musical experiences, and incorporating high and low intensity throughout a range of musical elements.

Musical decisions and judgments are based on the clinical situation in regards to the client's responses, developmental level, and interests.

If the client does not exhibit the target response after several musical attempts, it is recommended that supportive interventions (i.e., verbal, visual, and physical) be incorporated into the musical-play. (See Chapter 2 regarding procedures for providing supportive interventions.)

Clinical techniques

Assessing musical affect involves the implantation of clinical techniques that are focused on meeting the client's affect, evoking affective responses, and redirecting the client's attention. Therefore, the following techniques should be incorporated into musical-play: imitating, synchronizing, incorporating, pacing, reflecting, exaggerating, rhythmic grounding, tonal centering, holding, sharing instruments, giving, bonding, repeating, making spaces, interjecting, extending, and/or completing (Bruscia, 1987).

Considerations

In addition to observing target responses of musical affect, the therapist should consider the client's preferences and individual differences that may be interfering with his/her ability to express musical affect. The following questions should be considered during clinical observations/listening:

- Does the client display an increase in affect during particular musical contexts or arrangements?

- Is the client's affect impacted when the therapist incorporates verbal or nonverbal singing?

- Is the client's expression of affect congruent to the musical experience at hand?

- Does the client display the ability to socially reference the therapist in musical-play and if so, is it related to the musical experience?

- Does the client's musical response display emotional or expressive qualities (e.g., prosody when vocalizing, dynamic or tempo changes, etc.) that are congruent with the musical experience?

Level III: Adaption to Musical-Play

Adapting to the environment is the most important concept in human functioning (Piaget, 1962; Piaget & Barbel, 1969). When adapting, the individual is engaged in a continuous process of using the environment to learn, while learning to adjust to changes in the environment (Piaget, 1962). The music therapy process is no different. Adapting to various musical contexts involves experiences in which the client is actively learning new ways of relating and communicating in musical-play by following the therapist's lead, while adapting accordingly.

Through the process of modifying and adapting in musical-play the client is making adjustments that involve sustaining musical readiness, relatedness, and mutuality. He/she is intentionally making choices that are based on the moment-to-moment musical interactions that expand and change extemporaneously.

Adaption to musical-play deals with the client's ability to engage in a musical form of parallel play within the context of music making. The client follows what the therapist is doing as a play partner, but does not necessarily respond to specific musical elements. There are four areas of adaption to musical-play that the therapist is evaluating:

- Join: how the client enters into musical-play as led by therapist.

- Adjust: how the client adapts self-participation in musical-play as led by therapist.

- Takes turns: how the client enters into alternating musical-play as led by therapist.

- Stop: how the client concludes musical-play when therapist stops.

Assessing Adaption to Musical-Play

Instructions

Musical experiences assessing adaption to musical-play involve the client following the therapist's lead. Therefore it is required that the therapist implements musical strategies that will cue the client based on the desired target response. This may include the use of exaggerating articulation and/or attack on a particular or combined group of instrument/s including the therapist's voice. It may also involve extending cadence chords to maintain tension and delay resolution, thereby directing the client's attention to the musical-play situation, while also letting the client know that the therapist is waiting for him/her to join into the play. Musical strategies that may evoke the client's capacity to adapt in musical-play involve incorporating a wide range of tempo and/or dynamic changes, and variations in rhythm or meter in order to assess if the client recognizes any alterations in the musical experience. Generally, any musical changes can provide the client with the opportunity to adjust his/her playing. These changes should be presented in a musically related manner so that they are connected to the original musical context and may be utilized as a way to interrupt the client's playing and redirect his/her music.

Musical forms that may provide for turn-taking opportunities include musical phrases that call for resolution or response (e.g., antiphonal musical experiences). Essentially, the therapist provides a musical space or opening for the client to enter, or the therapist provides a "call" phrase, in anticipation of the client's response. Such musical frameworks should be presented by incorporating repetition as well as a range of tempo, dynamics, attack, and articulation at the points of a desired musical response (means of cuing the client).

Musical techniques that cue the client of a musical ending include decreasing tempo and dynamics, clear cadence, rubato, and ritardando. In addition, harmonic changes such as chromatic movement leading to the I chord (tonic) or implanting diminished 7th and/or augmented chords may also evoke the client to bring his/her music to a stop.

In all of the musical interventions utilized, it is important that all experiences and strategies are presented within a particular musical context. If the target response is not evident after several musical attempts, it is recommended that supportive interventions (i.e., verbal, visual, and physical) be incorporated into the musical-play. (See Chapter 2 regarding procedures for providing supportive interventions.)

Clinical techniques

Clinical techniques used to elicit the client's capacity to adapt to musical-play should be focused on eliciting and redirecting musical responses, such as repeating, modeling, making space, completing, introducing change, differentiating, modulating, intensifying, calming, and/or intervening (Bruscia, 1987).

Considerations

In addition to observing and listening for target responses of adaption in musical-play, the therapist should consider the client's preferences and individual differences that may be interfering with his/her ability to adapt to musical-play. The following questions should be considered during clinical observations/listening:

- Does the client understand the purpose of a particular instrument and have the ability to play it?

- Does the client require modeling on a particular instrument for context and understanding?

- Does the client display with motor planning and sequencing challenges in musical-play?

- Does the client display the ability to receive or read and understand the musical cues being presented?

- Does the client display the ability to express or communicate a musical response in a related and reciprocal manner?

- Does the client display the ability to understand cause-and-effect relationships in musical-play?

Level IV: Musical Engagement

To be intentional and mutual in music making may imply that there is an awareness and understanding of the relational dynamics musically occurring between two individuals. Musical intentionality derives from a desire to be purposeful and meaningful within musical interactions while indicating a desire to relate (or not) and be a part of something larger than one's self.

Developing and presenting opportunities for musical engagement involves providing the client with explicit and clear musical cues. Whereby the previous music domain (adapting to music-play) emphasizes the client's ability to follow the therapist's cues as a play partner (parallel play) not specific to musical elements, musical engagement focuses on the client's ability to match and engage the therapist's music, specific to musical elements. Here, as in the previous music domain area, the client is following the therapist's musical lead and directly engaging in and with the therapist's music. Musical engagement is the first music domain area examining the client's ability to engage in parallel/interactive play.

Musical engagement deals with the client's ability to utilize specific musical elements to match and engage the therapist's music. It is a form of parallel and interactive play in which the client engages in the therapist's music as cued. There are four areas of musical engagement being examined:

- Imitates: echoes musical phrases as led by therapist.

- Synchronizes: matches musical elements of therapist's music (e.g., tempo, dynamic, etc.) as led by therapist.

- Predicts: anticipates recurring musical responses as led by therapist.

- Ends: provides musical endings as led by therapist.

Assessing Musical Engagement

Instructions

The instructions for this domain are quite similar to the previous (adapting to musical-play). The differences are based on the target responses in each of the categories.

A starting point may be to develop a clear and simple melody (based on the moment-to-moment interaction) that may or may not be accompanied by a chord structure (depending on the client and clinical situation). The melody may be introduced as a theme or motif and is repeated in either its original or varied form. After a theme has been developed, it is important to be mindful of the client's level of attention and connection to the theme in regards to the musical components.

Musical techniques that may provide opportunities for the client to demonstrate his/her ability to imitate and predict can include the use of repetition and musical space while providing musical consistency and stability in dynamic and tempo.

Developing a clear musical structure and form may facilitate the client's ability to synchronize (e.g., music experiences that maintain a basic beat while accenting on the strong beats such as the second and fourth beats in 4/4 time). In addition, musical endings may be indicated by decreasing tempo and dynamics, offering a clear cadence, altering the harmony, and implementing rubato and/or ritardando.

If the target response is not observed after several musical attempts, supportive interventions (i.e., verbal, visual, and physical) may be incorporated into the musical-play. (See Chapter 2 regarding procedures for providing supportive interventions.)

Clinical techniques

The focal point of the techniques used when examining capacities in the area of musical engagement should be on structuring and eliciting musical responses. They include rhythmic grounding, tonal centering, shaping, repeating, modeling, and making space (Bruscia, 1987).

Considerations

Observing target responses of musical engagement also includes examining the client's preferences and individual differences that may be interfering with his/her ability to musically engage. The following questions should be considered during clinical observations/listening:

- What may be impeding the client's ability to engage in relational music making?
    - Receptive or expressive difficulties?
    - Sensory processing challenges?
    - Challenges with motor planning and sequencing?
    - Visual processing difficulties?
- What are the musical qualities and range of the client's music making?
    - Is the client's music relational?
    - Can the client play and sustain a basic beat in a related fashion?
    - Does the client display the ability to maintain tempo and dynamic levels during musical-play that are related to the therapist?
    - At what tempo and dynamic level does the client appear to have difficulty in maintaining musical engagement and relatedness?
    - At what tempo and dynamic level is the client able to play freely, flexibly, and comfortably?
    - Are the musical interactions between the client and therapist fragmented or intermittent? (See Chapter 2 for quality of musical interactions.)

Level V: Musical Interrelatedness

Interrelating within a social context includes the ability to communicate and relate in a mutual and reciprocal manner. It involves the ability to seek out meaningful relationships and understand social dynamics and cues. Interrelating within a musical context is no different.

Musical interrelatedness deals with the client's ability to be creative, expressive, and communicative while engaged in related music making. In addition, it involves the client initiating musical ideas and changes while also being able to differentiate between his/her and the therapist's music. It also includes the capacity to connect, assimilate, and integrate musical ideas in a reciprocal manner. Finally, musical interrelatedness involves the client being able to independently initiate changes in leadership and follower roles during musical experiences. This domain area examines the client's ability to truly interact in musical-play by contributing his/her ideas to engage the therapist, whereas the first four music domain areas deal with the client attending and responding to the therapist's music. Interrelatedness also includes the client's ability to create ideas based on the therapist's and interchangeably take on the role of both leader and follower. Musical interrelatedness includes eight areas:

- Initiate: how the client spontaneously begins a meaningful musical interaction with intent to present a new idea to the therapist.

- Change: how the client spontaneously initiates meaningful and original changes in any musical element.

- Differentiate: how the client takes role of soloist or accompanist, using own musical material; contrasts own musical elements in relation to therapist.

- Assimilate: how the client incorporates therapist's musical ideas into own original music.

- Connect: how the client bridges original musical material to a phrase and section in a meaningful and contextual manner.

- Interject: how the client inserts original ideas into musical spaces of therapist.

- Complete: how the client uses own musical ideas to create closure to music.

- Lead/follow: how the client independently initiates changes in leadership and followership roles with therapist.

Assessing Musical Interrelatedness

Instructions

When evaluating musical interrelatedness it is important to recognize and interpret the intent of the client's musical ideas/action before offering a musical response. Musical interactions are led by the client and require supportive, reinforcing, and reflective musical strategies that are related and clearly connected to the client's original music. Eliciting the client's ability to initiate a musical interaction or change in musical material requires patience, active listening, and restraint from offering a musical idea until it has been determined that the client requires support and guidance.

Musical strategies to assess differentiation may include either musically separating from the client's music, or refraining from musically following the client when he/she initiates a musical change. Other strategies include soloing over the client's accompaniment, and/or leaving musical space for the client to solo.

Musical interventions that may promote assimilation on the part of the client may involve offering or interjecting a related, but original, musical idea into the interaction. This may include presenting a new musical part or a change in any of the musical components. The idea is to interject an original musical idea that is clear and simple enough for the client to incorporate in some form into his/her original music. Interjecting musical ideas on the part of the client can be elicited by offering the client musical space within a framework, providing the client with room to insert his/her idea into the musical experience.

Musical forms that provide the opportunity to complete a musical idea include the implementation of musical phrases that ask to be resolved or answered. These types of phrases may also include a decrease in tempo and dynamics in which the last beat or two are left off for the client to fill with music. The decrease in tempo and dynamics may indicate that an ending is nearing, while the omitting of the last beat or two provides the space for the client to complete the phrase.

Facilitating opportunities for the client to initiate role changes (lead and follow) may involve musical experiences that enhance the client's musical responses in order to extend and expand the play, as well as closing or answering phrases initiated by the client.

If the target response is not evident after several musical attempts, it is recommended that supportive interventions (i.e., verbal, visual, and physical) be incorporated into the musical-play. (See Chapter two regarding procedures for providing supportive interventions.)

Clinical techniques

The implementation of clinical techniques when assessing musical interrelatedness should focus on supporting the client's ability to initiate musical ideas by providing empathy, structure, and guidance. Any of the following techniques may be used: imitating, synchronizing, incorporating, pacing, reflecting, exaggerating, rhythmic grounding, tonal centering, shaping, sharing instruments, repeating, making spaces, interjecting, extending, and completing (Bruscia, 1987).

Considerations

It is suggested that the therapist focus his/her observation/listening on attempting to understand the client's musical desire and intent. The therapist should consider and determine the following:

- Can the client initiate and/or close (ending) circles of musical communication in a related manner? (See Chapter two for circles of communication.)

- Can the client engage in a continuous flow of reciprocal musical-play with the therapist?

- Can the client independently change between the role of leader and follower in musical-play, or can he/she only lead or only follow?

- Can the client maintain musical relatedness while differentiating music?

- Can the client initiate expressive components in musical-play (e.g., tempo changes, etc.) in a contextual, meaningful, and purposeful manner?

- Can the client maintain relatedness after initiating a musical change?

- Can the client initiate and express a range of musical changes in musical-play?

- Can the client integrate musical changes by joining and/or initiating them?

Scoring Instructions

The MEARS can be used descriptively to profile a client's musical responsiveness based on the five music domain areas. It can also be used quantitatively by rating each category of the domain areas. Scoring the MEARS involves the therapist observing target music responses as they are exhibited during the session or segment thereof. Several target music responses may be observed simultaneously depending on the client's abilities. Observations include the therapist rating the frequency of the target response, level of support provided for the target response, as well as indicating the medium in which the client offered the target response.

Frequency	*Support*
1 = exhibits musical response rarely if ever	1 = maximum (full physical)
2 = exhibits musical response occasionally	2 = moderate (partial physical)
3 = exhibits musical response about half of the time	3 = mild support (visual)
4 = exhibits musical response often but not always	4 = minimal (verbal)
5 = consistently exhibits musical response	5 = no support (independent)

Media

I = Instrumental, V = Vocal, and M = Movement

Rating scores for each variable, i.e., frequency and support, can be added together and divided by the amount of categories (target responses) in order to calculate total average scores for each domain area. Rating scores for level of support should indicate the highest level provided for the target response. Total average scores (sub scores) are then interpreted by using the frequency scale and level of support scale. In addition, all of the media in which the client offered target responses should be indicated in the "total" box. (See Figure 6.)

Figure 6. Scoring example of MEARS

I. MUSICAL ATTENTION	Frequency	Support	Media
a) Focuses	2	3	I,M
b) Maintains	2	3	I,M
c) Shares	1	2	I,V,M
d) Shifts	1	2	I,V.M
Total/Avg.	6/1.5	10/2.5	I,V,M

II. MUSICAL AFFECT	Frequency	Support	Media
e) Facial	3	3	I
f) Prosody	1	3	V
g) Body	2	2	I,M
h) Motion	2	2	I,M
Total/Avg.	8/2	10/2.5	I,V,M

Analyzing and Interpreting Scores

The MEARS scoring example in Figure 6 examined the client's ability to musically attend (musical attention) and respond affectively (musical affect) in musical-play. The rating scores in "musical attention" include a "2" (exhibits musical response occasionally) in the frequency row and a "3" (mild support) in the support row under the columns of "focus" and "maintains" when the client was engaged in instrument play and movement. The client also scored a rating of "1" (exhibits musical response rarely if ever) in the frequency row and a "2" (moderate support) in the support row under the columns of "shares" and "shifts" when engaged in instrument play, vocalizing (singing), and movement in musical-play. Thus, the client's overall total average scores (sub scores) in the area of musical attention include a rating score of "1.5" (exhibits musical response occasionally) in the frequency row and a "2.5" (mild support) in the support row. The total media in which the client offered target responses in the area of musical attention are instrumental, vocal, and movement.

The rating scores in the area of musical affect indicate a "3" (exhibits musical response about half of the time) in the frequency row and a "3" (mild support) in the support row under the column of "facial" when the client was engaged in instrument play. The client also scored a rating of "1" (exhibits musical response rarely if ever) in the frequency row and a "3" (mild support) in the support row under the column of "prosody" when vocalizing (singing) in musical-play. In addition, the client scored a rating of "2" (exhibits musical response occasionally) in the frequency row and a "2" (moderate support) in the support row under the columns of "body" and "motion" when engaged in instrumental play and movement. Hence, the client's overall total average score (sub score) in the area of musical affect include a rating score of "2" (exhibits musical response occasionally) in the frequency row and a "2.5" (mild support) in the support row. The total media in which the client offered target responses in the area of musical affect are instrumental, vocal, and movement.

Chapter 4 — Scale II: Musical Cognitive/Perception Scale

Summary of Chapter

Chapter 4 presents the Musical Cognition/Perception Scale (MCPS). The chapter includes a detailed description of the MCPS, criteria of target responses, protocols and procedures, clinical techniques, considerations, and scoring instructions. The MCPS examines the client's ability to react, focus, recall, follow and initiate rhythm, melody, dynamic, phrase, and timbre in musical-play. Scoring is based on frequency of response and media in which the client offered the response. (See Figure 7.)

Figure 7. Example of the MCPS evaluting the client's ability to react and focus in musical-play

	Rhythm	Melody	Dynamic	Phrase	Timbre	Total/Avg.
Reacts	I/5; V/5	I/5; V/5	I/3; M/4	I/2	V/2	**31/3.87**
Focuses	I/4;V/3	V/3	I/3	I/1	V/2	**16/2.6**

The Musical Cognitive/Perception Scale (MCPS)

The Musical Cognitive/Perception Scale (MCPS) is a criterion-referenced instrument designed to assess and evaluate the client's musical cognitive/perceptual skills in musical-play based on five areas: 1) *react*, 2) *focus*, 3) *recall*, 4) *follow*, and 5) *initiate*. Each of the five areas is evaluated based on five specific musical elements: 1) rhythm, 2) melody, 3) dynamic, 4) phrasing, and 5) timbre.

The MCPS was developed as a means to understand the mental processes that support musical behaviors involved in relational music making including awareness, comprehension, memory, attention, and performance. In addition, it was designed for music therapists to attain an understanding of the client's musical sensitivity in musical-play, including sensitivity to relational rather than absolute properties of rhythm, melody, dynamics, phrasing, and timbre.

The four cognitive/perceptual areas are informed by music cognition (Levitin, 2006; Patel, 2010; Honing, 2012) as well as the author's task analysis (Carpente, 2009, 2011, 2012) that are pertinent to neurodevelopmental disorders.

Area I: Reacts

Reacts deals with how the client responds affectively or behaviorally to each of the five musical elements: rhythm, melody, dynamic, phrasing, and timbre. This involves any active musical response on the part of the client in any of the three media (i.e. vocal, movement, and/or instrument) that is related to the musical experience. This may include the client responding via a gesture, an utterance, expressing on an instrument, vocally, and/or via movement.

Evaluating the client's ability to react to musical elements begins by closely observing and listening to the client through various musical experiences within the context of related music making. Observations and listening are based on how the client reacts (target response) to a particular element and the frequency in which the client reacts to the element in musical-play.

Observation and listening

Rhythm

To what extent can the client react to rhythmic elements (i.e., pulse, tempo, meter, patterns, and/or subdivisions) and changes therein in musical-play? More specifically, how frequently and through which media does the client exhibit the ability to react to rhythmic elements in musical-play?

Melody

To what extent can the client react to elements of melody (i.e., direction, key, tonality, and/or steps) and changes therein in musical-play? More specifically, how frequently and through which media does the client demonstrate the ability to react to elements of melody in musical-play?

Dynamic

To what extent can the client react to dynamic (loud and soft) and changes therein in musical-play? More specifically, how frequently and through which media does the client display the ability to react to dynamic in musical-play?

Phrase

To what extent can the client react to musical phrasing (i.e., length, shape, articulation, and expression) and changes therein in musical-play? More specifically, how frequently and through which media does the client exhibit the ability to react to musical phrasing in musical-play?

Timbre

To what extent can the client react to timbre (i.e., sound quality, including resonance, attack, articulation, and/or expression) and changes therein in musical-play? More specifically, how frequently and through which media does the client demonstrate the ability to react to timbre in musical-play?

Clinical techniques

Clinical techniques used to assess and evaluate the client's ability to react include repeating, modeling, making space, completing, introducing change, differentiating, modulating, intensifying, calming, and intervening (Bruscia, 1987).

Considerations

The following questions should be considered when assessing and evaluating the client's ability to react to musical elements in musical-play:

- Does a particular musical media being played by the therapist and/or client impact the client's ability to react to an element in musical-play?

- Does a particular musical context, element/s and/or arrangement impact the client's ability to react to an element in musical-play?

- Is the client's ability to react to an element in musical-play impacted by the therapist incorporating verbal or nonverbal singing?

- Does the client display a range in his ability to react to an element in musical-play?

- Does the client react in a hyper/ and/or hyporeactive manner to an element in musical-play?

- Does the client react reflexively and/or intentionally to an element in musical-play?

- Does the client react to an element in musical-play to fulfill a sensory need or is it purely musical (relational)?

- Does the environment (e.g., lighting, objects in the room, etc.) impact the client's ability to react to an element in musical-play?

- Does the client react to particular musical scenarios, elements, and/or media by engaging in self-perseverative behaviors in musical-play? If so, are the perseverative behaviors related to the music in any way?

- Does the client react to particular musical scenarios, elements, and/or media in a destructive or harmful manner?

- Can the client maintain self-regulation when reacting to an element in musical-play?

- Are there any recognizable patterns to when and how the client reacts to an element in musical-play?

- Does the client require supportive interventions in order to demonstrate the ability to react to an element in musical-play?

Area II: Focus

Focus refers to how the client attends to musical elements as led by the therapist. This involves the client's ability to sustain readiness, calmness, and alertness while monitoring impulses in musical-play. Evaluation is based on observing and listening to the client's focus of attention on each the five musical elements in musical-play.

Observation and listening

Rhythm

To what extent can the client focus attention on rhythmic elements (i.e., pulse, tempo, meter, patterns and/or subdivisions) and changes therein in musical-play? More specifically, how frequently and through which media does the client display the ability to focus attention to rhythmic elements in musical-play?

Melody

To what extent can the client focus attention to elements of melody (i.e., direction, key, tonality, and/or steps) and changes therein in musical-play? More specifically, how frequently and via which media does the client exhibit the ability to focus attention on elements of melody in musical-play?

Dynamic

To what extent can the client focus attention on dynamic (loud and soft) and changes therein in musical-play? More specifically, how frequently and through which media does the client exhibit the ability to focus attention on dynamic in musical-play?

Phrase

To what extent can the client focus attention to musical phrasing (i.e., length, shape, articulation, and expression) and changes therein in musical-play? More specifically, how frequently and through which media does the client focus attention to musical phrasing in musical-play?

Timbre

To what extent can the client focus attention on timbre (i.e., sound quality, including resonance, attack, articulation, and/or expression) and changes therein in musical-play? More specifically, how frequently and through which media does the client exhibit the ability to focus attention on timbre in musical-play?

Clinical techniques

Clinical techniques used to assess and evaluate the client's ability to focus include imitating, synchronizing, incorporating, pacing, reflecting, exaggerating, rhythmic grounding, tonal centering, sharing instruments, repeating, making spaces, extending, and completing (Bruscia, 1987).

Considerations

The following questions should be considered when assessing and evaluating the client's ability to focus attention to music elements in musical-play:

- What elements or combination of elements does the client display attentional focus to in musical-play?

- Does the client display attentional focus to an element in musical-play when a particular combination of media is being used?

- Does the client display attentional focus to an element in musical-play when playing a percussive instrument that requires the use of mallets?

- Does the client display attentional focus to an element in musical-play when playing percussion instruments that require the use of hands and/or feet?

- Is the client's ability to sustain attentional focus to an element in musical-play impacted by his/her individual differences, such as poor gait and balance, low muscle tone, poor motor planning and sequencing, and/or difficulties with sensory processing and/or visual spatial capacities?

- Is the client's ability to sustain attentional focus to an element in musical-play impacted by his/her ability to maintain self-regulation?

- Does the client require supportive interventions in order to display attentional focus to an element in musical-play?

Area III: Recall

Recall refers to the client's ability to display recognition of repeated musical patterns by imitating, predicting, and/or ending the therapist's music. Repeated musical patterns may include a melodic shape or phrase, a melodic rhythm, a sequence in dynamic, and/or a sequence that involves a change in timbre.

Observation and listening

Rhythm

To what extent can the client recall a rhythmic pattern in musical-play? More specifically, how frequently and through which media does the client exhibit his/her ability to recall a rhythmic pattern in musical-play?

Melody

To what extent can the client recall a melodic pattern in musical-play? More specifically, how frequently and through which media does the client display the ability to recall a melodic pattern in musical-play?

Dynamic

To what extent can the client recall a dynamic pattern in musical-play? More specifically, how frequently and through which media does the client demonstrate the ability to recall a dynamic pattern in musical-play?

Phrase

To what extent can the client recall a repeated musical phrase in musical-play? More specifically, how frequently and through which media does the client display the ability to recall a musical phrase in musical-play?

Timbre

To what extent can the client recall timbre in musical-play? More specifically, how frequently and through which media does the client display the ability to recall timbre in musical-play?

Clinical techniques

Clinical techniques used to assess and evaluate the client's ability to recall include rhythmic grounding, tonal centering, shaping, repeating, modeling, and making space (Bruscia, 1987).

Considerations

The following questions should be considered when evaluating and assessing the client's ability to recall musical elements in musical-play:

- Does the client display the ability to anticipate repeated musical patterns in musical-play?

- Does the client display the ability to recall particular musical patterns, elements, and/or contexts in musical-play?

- Does the client display the ability to recall an element in musical-play through a range of musical contexts and music experiences?

- Does the client display the ability to recall an element in musical-play when playing a particular media?

- Does the client display the ability to recall an element in musical-play when the therapist is playing a particular media?

- Does the client display the ability to recall an element and musical patterns in musical-play from session to session?

- Does the client require supportive interventions in order to display the ability to recall an element in musical-play?

Area IV: Follow

Follow refers to the client's ability to change a musical element in order to match the therapist's music and/or how the client follows the therapist in regards to specific musical elements. This may include how the client follows the therapist's music in terms of changes to rhythmic elements, melody, dynamics, phrasing, or timbre.

Observation and listening

Rhythm

To what extent can the client follow a rhythmic change in musical-play? More specifically, how frequently and through which media does the client exhibit the ability to follow a rhythmic change in musical-play?

Melody

To what extent can the client follow a change of melody in musical-play? More specifically, how frequently and through which media does the client exhibit the ability to follow a change in melody in musical-play?

Dynamic

To what extent can the client follow a change of dynamic in musical-play? More specifically, how frequently and through which media does the client display the ability to follow a change of dynamic in musical-play?

Phrase

To what extent can the client follow a change of phrasing in musical-play? More specifically, how frequently and through which media does the client demonstrate the ability to follow a change of phrasing in musical-play?

Timbre

To what extent can the client follow a change of timbre in musical-play? More specifically, how frequently and through which media does the client display the ability to follow a change of timbre in musical-play?

Clinical techniques

Clinical techniques used to assess and evaluate the client's ability to follow changes to musical elements include repeating, modeling, making space, completing, introducing change, differentiating, modulating, intensifying, calming, and intervening (Bruscia, 1987).

Considerations

The following questions should be considered when assessing and evaluating the client's ability to follow changes of elements in musical-play:

- Does the client display the ability to follow changes of musical elements in musical-play through a range of musical scenarios, elements, and/or contexts?

- Is the client's ability to follow changes of musical elements in musical-play solely based on a stimulus-response way of responding or is it based on a desire to be musically related?

- Does the client require supportive interventions in order to display the ability to follow changes of musical elements in musical-play?

Area V: Initiate

Initiate refers to the client's ability to spontaneously manipulate a musical element in a related and contextual manner in musical-play. This may include the client initiating a change in rhythm, melody, dynamic, phrasing, and/or timbre.

Observation and listening

Rhythm

To what extent can the client spontaneously manipulate (initiate) a rhythmic element in musical-play? More specifically, how frequently and through which media does the client exhibit the ability to spontaneously manipulate (initiate) a rhythmic element in musical-play?

Melody

To what extent can the client spontaneously manipulate (initiate) melody in musical-play? More specifically, how frequently and through which media does the client exhibit the ability to spontaneously manipulate (initiate) melody in musical-play?

Dynamic

To what extent can the client spontaneously manipulate (initiate) dynamic in musical-play? More specifically, how frequently and through which media does the client display the ability to spontaneously manipulate (initiate) dynamic in musical-play?

Phrase

To what extent can the client spontaneously manipulate (initiate) phrasing in musical-play? More specifically, how frequently and through which media does the client demonstrate the ability to spontaneously manipulate (initiate) phrasing in musical-play?

Timbre

To what extent can the client spontaneously manipulate (initiate) timbre in musical-play? More specifically, how frequently and through which media does the client display the ability to spontaneously manipulate (initiate) timbre in musical-play?

Clinical techniques

Clinical techniques used to assess and evaluate the client's ability to spontaneously manipulate (initiate) musical elements in musical-play include imitating, synchronizing, incorporating, pacing, reflecting, exaggerating, rhythmic grounding, tonal centering, shaping, sharing instruments, repeating, making spaces, interjecting, extending, and completing (Bruscia, 1987).

Considerations

The following questions should be considered when assessing and evaluating the client's ability to spontaneously manipulate (initiate) a musical element in musical-play:

- Does the client spontaneously manipulate (initiate) an element in musical-play for the purpose of relating and/or communicating or is it based on fulfilling a sensory need?

- Does the client spontaneously manipulate (initiate) an element in musical-play for the purpose of seeking out the therapist's music?

- Does the client generally need to initiate a change in an element; does he/she become agitated when initiating a musical idea?

- Does the client display the ability to spontaneously manipulate (initiate) an element in musical-play through a range of musical scenarios, elements, and/or contexts; does he/she only initiate during specific types of musical experiences and contexts?

- Does the client require supportive interventions in order to display the ability to spontaneously manipulate (initiate) an element in musical-play?

Chapter 4: Scale II: Musical Cognitive/Perception Scale

Scoring Instructions

The MCPS can be used descriptively to profile a client's musical cognitive/perceptual skills in musical-play. It can also be used quantitatively by rating each category of the musical cognitive/perceptual areas.

Scoring the MCPS involves the therapist observing target music responses as they are displayed during the session or segment thereof. Several target music responses may be observed simultaneously depending on the client's abilities. Observations include the therapist rating the frequency of the target response as well as indicating the media in which the client offered the target response.

Frequency

1 = exhibits musical response rarely if ever

2 = exhibits musical response occasionally

3 = exhibits musical response about half of the time

4 = exhibits musical response often but not always

5 = consistently exhibits musical response

Media

I = Instrumental, V = Vocal, and M = Movement

Rating scores for each frequency variable can be added together and divided by the amount of frequency rating scores in a particular category (music target response) in order to calculate average scores for each category. Average scores for each target music response category are then interpreted by using the frequency response scale. (See Figure 8.)

Figure 8. Scoring example of the MCPS

	Rhythm	Melody	Dynamic	Phrase	Timbre	Total/Avg.
Follows	I/1; M/1	I/1	I/2	I/2	I/2	9/1.5
Initiates	I/2	I/2	I/1	I/1	I/1;V/1	8/1.33

Analyzing and Interpreting Scores

The MCPS scoring example in Figure 8 examined the client's ability to "follow" and "initiate" rhythm, melody, dynamic, phrasing, and timbre in musical-play.

The scoring example indicates a rating score of "1" (exhibits musical response rarely if ever) in regards to "follows" rhythm when engaged in instrument play and movement. In addition, the client scored a rating of "1" in regards to "follows" melody when playing an instrument in musical-play and a rating score of "2" (exhibits musical response occasionally) pertaining to "follows" dynamic, phrase, and timbre when playing an instrument in musical-play. Thus, the client's overall total average score (sub score) in the area of "follows" is "1.5" (exhibits musical response rarely if ever).

In the area of "initiates" the client scored a rating of "2" pertaining to "initiates" rhythm and melody when playing an instrument in musical-play and a rating score of "1" in regards to "initiates" dynamic and phrase when playing an instrument in musical-play. Finally, the client scored a rating of "1" in regards to "initiates" timbre when vocalizing (singing) and engaging in instrument play. Hence, the client's overall total average score (sub score) in the area of "initiates" is "1.33" (exhibits musical response rarely if ever).

CHAPTER 5 SCALE III: MUSICAL RESPONSIVENESS SCALE

Summary of Chapter

Chapter 5 introduces the Musical Responsiveness Scale (MRS). The chapter includes a detailed description of the MRS, criteria of target responses, protocols and procedures, clinical techniques, considerations, and scoring instructions. The MRS examines the client's overall responsiveness in musical-play specifically in the areas of musical preferences, perceptual efficiency, and self-regulation through the ranges of tempo, dynamics, pitch, and attack in each of the three media (instruments, vocal, and movement) in musical-play. Scoring is based on frequency of the target music response. (See Figure 9.)

Figure 9. Example of the MRS evaluating the client's overall responsiveness when vocalizing in musical-play.

		TEMPO RANGE			DYN. RANGE			PITCH RANGE			ATTACK		
		Slow	Med	Fast	Soft	Med	Loud	Low	Mid	High	PS	SL	PL
V O C A L	Preference	1	1	1	3	1	3	1	3	1	3	1	1
	Efficiency	1	1	1	3	1	3	1	3	1	3	1	1
	Self-Regulation	1-	1-	1-	3	1-	3	1-	3	1-	3	1	1

The Musical Responsiveness Scale (MRS)

The Musical Responsiveness Scale (MRS) is a criterion-based instrument designed to assess and evaluate the overall responses and tendencies of the client at the various ranges of tempo, dynamics, pitch, and attack in musical-play based on three areas: 1) *preferences*, 2) *perceptual efficiency* and 3) *self-regulation*. Each area is assessed in each of the three media i.e., voice, instrument, and movement.

The MRS was developed for music therapists to identify their clients preferences, motivations, and efficiency as well as their ability to self-regulate in musical-play. It can also be used to recognize relationships between the three areas (i.e., preferences, perceptual efficiency, and self-regulation) and serve as a musical guide to inform the therapist's music.

Area I: Preferences

Preferences for a particular range of a musical element can be reflexive, learned through exposure or conditioning, and/or intentional. It is not skill related. It is, however, affective-based. The preference section of the scale provides the motivational substratum for perceptual efficiency. Hence, preferences deal with the extent to which the client responds with positive affect in a particular media, i.e., vocal, instrumental, and movement.

Observation: Preferences/vocal

Tempo range

To what extent does the client respond vocally with positive affect in regard to tempo range in musical-play? More specifically, how frequently does the client respond vocally with positive affect within a particular tempo range in musical-play?

Dynamic range

To what extent does the client respond vocally with positive affect in regard to dynamic range in musical-play? More specifically, how frequently does the client respond vocally with positive affect within a particular dynamic range in musical-play?

Pitch range

To what extent does the client respond vocally with positive affect in regard to pitch range in musical-play? More specifically, how frequently does the client respond vocally with positive affect within a particular pitch range in musical-play?

Attack range

To what extent does the client respond vocally with positive affect in regard to range of attack in musical-play? More specifically, how frequently does the client respond vocally with positive affect within a particular range of attack in musical-play?

Observation: Preferences/instrument

Tempo range

To what extent does the client respond instrumentally with positive affect in regard to tempo range in musical-play? More specifically, how frequently does the client respond instrumentally with positive affect within a tempo range in musical-play?

Dynamic range

To what extent does the client respond instrumentally with positive affect in regard to dynamic range in musical-play? More specifically, how frequently does the client respond instrumentally with positive affect within a particular dynamic range in musical-play?

Pitch range

To what extent does the client respond instrumentally with positive affect in regard to pitch range in musical-play? More specifically, how frequently does the client respond instrumentally with positive affect within a particular pitch range in musical-play?

Attack range

To what extent does the client respond instrumentally with positive affect in regard to range of attack in musical-play? More specifically, how frequently does the client respond instrumentally with positive affect within a particular range of attack in musical-play?

Observation: Preferences/movement

Tempo range

To what extent does the client respond through movement with positive affect in regard to tempo range in musical-play? More specifically, how frequently does the client respond through movement with positive affect within a particular tempo range in musical-play?

Dynamic range

To what extent does the client respond through movement with positive affect in regard to dynamic range in musical-play? More specifically, how frequently does the client respond through movement with positive affect within a particular dynamic range in musical-play?

Pitch range

To what extent does the client respond through movement with positive affect in regard to pitch range in musical-play? More specifically, how frequently does the client respond through movement with positive affect within a particular pitch range in musical-play?

Attack range

To what extent does the client respond through movement with positive affect in regard to range of attack in musical-play? More specifically, how frequently does the client respond through movement with positive affect within a particular range of attack in musical-play?

Clinical techniques

Clinical techniques used to assess and evaluate the client's preferences include imitating, synchronizing, incorporating, pacing, reflecting, exaggerating, rhythmic grounding, tonal centering, holding, sharing instruments, giving, bonding, repeating, making spaces, interjecting, extending, and/or completing (Bruscia, 1987).

Considerations

The following questions should be considered during clinical observation/listening in musical-play, as well as during scoring:

- What is the client's most and least preferred musical scenario/s, element/s, combination of elements, and/or contexts?

- How does the client respond (e.g., dysregulated, withdraw from interaction) to most and least preferred musical scenario/s, element/s, combination of elements, and/or contexts?

- Does the client display a range of musical preferences?

- Does the client present with a pattern in regard to range of musical preferences (e.g., fast tempo and loud dynamic)?

- What is the client's least and most preferred media?

- What is the client's range of playing when engaged in his/her preferred media?

- What is the client's range of playing within his/her preferred musical preferences?

- Can the client maintain engagement when playing within his/her musical preferences in a continuous flowing manner?

- Does the client engage in musical-play within his/her musical preferences in a relational manner or are responses based on stimulus-response and/or sensory seeking?

Area II: Perceptual Efficiency

Perceptual efficiency within a particular range of a musical element may be innate or developmental. It is skill or talent related and reflects how well the client is able to manipulate the element given the preferences and motivations measured in the preference section of the scale. Thus, perceptual efficiency deals with the relative success the client has in a particular media (i.e., voice, instrument, and movement) when performing perceptual tasks.

Observation: Perceptual efficiency/vocal

Tempo range

To what extent is the client relatively successful, vocally, when performing perceptual tasks in regard to tempo range in musical-play? More specifically, how frequently successful is the client, vocally, when performing perceptual tasks in regard to tempo range in musical-play?

Dynamic range

To what extent is the client relatively successful, vocally, when performing perceptual tasks in regard to dynamic range in musical-play? More specifically, how frequently successful is the client, vocally, when performing perceptual tasks in regard to dynamic range in musical-play?

Pitch range

To what extent is the client relatively successful, vocally, when performing perceptual tasks in regard to pitch range in musical-play? More specifically, how frequently successful is the client, vocally, when performing perceptual tasks in regard to pitch range in musical-play?

Attack range

To what extent is the client relatively successful, vocally, when performing perceptual tasks in regard to range of attack in musical-play? More specifically, how frequently successful is the client, vocally, when performing perceptual tasks in regard to range of attack in musical-play?

Observation: Perceptual efficiency/instrument

Tempo range

To what extent is the client relatively successful, instrumentally, when performing perceptual tasks in regard to tempo range in musical-play? More specifically, how frequently successful is the client, instrumentally, when performing perceptual tasks in regard to tempo range in musical-play?

Dynamic range

To what extent is the client relatively successful, instrumentally, when performing perceptual tasks in regard to dynamic range in musical-play? More specifically, how frequently successful is the client, instrumentally, when performing perceptual tasks in regard to dynamic range in musical-play?

Pitch range

To what extent is the client relatively successful, instrumentally, when performing perceptual tasks in regard to pitch range in musical-play? More specifically, how frequently successful is the client, instrumentally, when performing perceptual tasks in regard to pitch range in musical-play?

Attack range

To what extent is the client relatively successful, instrumentally, when performing perceptual tasks in regard to range of attack in musical-play? More specifically, how frequently successful is the client, instrumentally, when performing perceptual tasks in regard to range of attack in musical-play?

Observation: Perceptual efficiency/movement

Tempo range

To what extent is the client relatively successful via movement when performing perceptual tasks in regard to tempo range in musical-play? More specifically, how frequently successful is the client via movement when performing perceptual tasks in regard to tempo range in musical-play?

Dynamic range

To what extent is the client relatively successful via movement when performing perceptual tasks in regard to dynamic range in musical-play? More specifically, how frequently successful is the client via movement when performing perceptual tasks in regard to dynamic range in musical-play?

Pitch range

To what extent is the client relatively successful via movement when performing perceptual tasks in regard to pitch range in musical-play? More specifically, how frequently successful is the client via movement when performing perceptual tasks in regard to pitch range in musical-play?

Attack range

To what extent is the client relatively successful via movement when performing perceptual tasks in regard to range of attack in musical-play? More specifically, how frequently successful is the client via movement when performing perceptual tasks in regard to range of attack in musical-play?

Clinical techniques

Clinical techniques used to assess and evaluate the client's perceptual efficiency include repeating, modeling, making space, completing, introducing change, differentiating, modulating, intensifying, calming, intervening, rhythmic grounding, tonal centering, and shaping (Bruscia, 1987).

Considerations

The following questions should be considered during clinical observation/listening in musical-play, as well as during scoring:

- Through which type of musical experience, musical elements, and contexts does the client display most and least perceptual efficiency?

- Can the client display perceptual efficiency in musical-play though a range of musical experiences and contexts?

- Does the client display greater perceptual efficiency when engaged in instrument play, and/or vocal play, and/or movement?

- Does the client maintain perceptual efficacy in a continuous flowing manner when engaged in musical-play?

- Does the client display perceptual efficiency in a relational manner or are responses based on stimulus-response and/or sensory-seeking responses?

Area III: Self-Regulation

Self-regulation within a particular range of a musical element is developmental. It reflects how well the client is able to manipulate a musical element given his/her ability to physically and emotionally control and manage impulses while sustaining focus and attention to the task at hand. Self-regulation deals with the extent to which the client maintains attention and availability for interaction and to musical elements while engaged within a particular media (i.e., voice, instrument, and movement) in musical-play.

Observation: Self-regulation/vocal

Tempo range

To what extent can the client sustain self-regulation while vocalizing in regard to tempo range in musical-play? More specifically, how frequently can the client sustain self-regulation while vocalizing in regard to tempo range in musical-play?

Dynamic Range

To what extent can the client sustain self-regulation while vocalizing in regard to dynamic range in musical-play? More specifically, how frequently can the client sustain self-regulation while vocalizing in regard to dynamic range in musical-play?

Pitch range

To what extent can the client sustain self-regulation while vocalizing in regard to pitch range in musical-play? More specifically, how frequently can the client sustain self-regulation while vocalizing in regard to pitch range in musical-play?

Attack range

To what extent can the client sustain self-regulation while vocalizing in regard to range of attack in musical-play? More specifically, how frequently can the client sustain self-regulation while vocalizing in regard to range of attack in musical-play?

Observation: Self-regulation/instrument

Tempo range

To what extent can the client sustain self-regulation while playing an instrument in regard to tempo range in musical-play? More specifically, how frequently can the client sustain self-regulation while playing an instrument in regard to tempo range in musical-play?

Dynamic Range

To what extent can the client sustain self-regulation while playing an instrument in regard to dynamic range in musical-play? More specifically, how frequently can the client sustain self-regulation while playing an instrument in regard to dynamic range in musical-play?

Pitch range

To what extent can the client sustain self-regulation while playing an instrument in regard to pitch range in musical-play? More specifically, how frequently can the client sustain self-regulation while playing an instrument in regard to pitch range in musical-play?

Attack range

To what extent can the client sustain self-regulation while playing an instrument in regard to range of attack in musical-play? More specifically, how frequently can the client sustain self-regulation while playing an instrument in regard to range of attack in musical-play?

Observation: Self-regulation/movement

Tempo range

To what extent can the client sustain self-regulation while engaged in movement in regard to tempo range in musical-play? More specifically, how frequently can the client sustain self-regulation while engaged in movement in regard to tempo range in musical-play?

Dynamic range

To what extent can the client sustain self-regulation while engaged in movement in regard to dynamic range in musical-play? More specifically, how frequently can the client sustain self-regulation while engaged in movement in regard to dynamic range in musical-play?

Pitch range

To what extent can the client sustain self-regulation while engaged in movement in regard to pitch range in musical-play? More specifically, how frequently can the client sustain self-regulation while engaged in movement in regard to pitch range in musical-play?

Attack range

To what extent can the client sustain self-regulation while engaged in movement in regard to range of attack in musical-play? More specifically, how frequently can the client sustain self-regulation while engaged in movement in regard to range of attack in musical-play?

Clinical techniques

Clinical techniques used to assess and evaluate the client's ability to self-regulate include imitating, synchronizing, incorporating, pacing, reflecting, exaggerating, rhythmic grounding, tonal centering, sharing instruments, repeating, making spaces, extending, and completing (Bruscia, 1987).

Considerations

The following questions should be considered when assessing and evaluating the client's ability to self-regulate:

- When does the client appear to get distressed?
- Where is the client's focus?
- What may the client's body language be saying?
- Does the client appear to be under-/ or overstimulated?
- Does the client have a look of fear?
- Is the client attentive to the music and/or to the therapist?
- Is the client experiencing sensory "overload" in terms to processing the music and/or other sensory information in the environment?
- Does the client "crave" movement?
   - Walking back and forth in a line?
   - Walking in circular motion?
   - Jumping up and down?
- What is the client's preferred self-stimulatory behavior/s?
- Are the client's self-stimulatory behaviors related to the music in any way (e.g., tempo, tonality, etc.)?
- What sensory needs are the self-stimulatory behaviors meeting (e.g., visual, tactile, vestibular, etc.)?
- Is the client under-/ or overreactive to the music experience?
   - What type of musical support may the client need to become "up-regulated" (e.g., music with increased dynamics, dissonance, high register, etc.)?
   - What type of nonmusical support may the client need in order to self-regulate (e.g., deep pressure, high affect through gestures, etc.)?
- Does the client display with mixed reactivity (over and underreactivity) to the music experience?

- How many consecutive measures is the client able to maintain self-regulation?
    - During receptive musical experiences?
    - During musical interactive experiences?
        - Simultaneous play?
        - Call-and-response?

Scoring Instructions

The MRS can be used descriptively to profile a client's overall preferences, perceptual efficiency, and self-regulation displayed throughout the session or segment therein. Scoring the MRS involves the therapist observing the overall tendencies of the client at different ranges of tempo, dynamics, pitch, and attack using the frequency rating scale. When scoring self-regulation add a "+" for hyperreactive, or a "-" for hyporeactive, or a "±" to indicate mixed reactivity. Thus, for example, "2 +" in the "fast tempo" row under "instrument" column signifies that the client is occasionally self-regulated and dysregulates in a hyperreactive manner during fast tempo music when engaged in instrument play. (See Figure 10.)

Target music responses may be observed simultaneously depending on the client's abilities. Observations include the therapist rating the frequency of response as well as indicating the media in which the client offered the response in musical-play.

Frequency

1 = exhibits musical response rarely if ever

2 = exhibits musical response occasionally

3 = exhibits musical response about half of the time

4 = exhibits musical response often but not always

5 = consistently exhibits musical response

Ranges of musical elements

a) <u>Tempi</u>: slow (adagio) = 66–76 bpm; medium (andante) = 76–108 bpm;

   fast (allegro) = 120–168 bpm

b) <u>Dynamics</u>: soft = piano; medium = mezzo-forte; loud = forte

c) <u>Pitch</u>: low = C3–B3; mid-range = C4–B4; high = C5–B5

d) <u>Attack</u>: PS = primarily staccato; SL= staccato and legato; PL= primarily legato

Rating scores of target music responses for the MRS are not computed. Each rating score is interpreted by using the frequency response scale.

Figure 10. Scoring example of the MRS

		TEMPO RANGE			DYN. RANGE			PITCH RANGE			ATTACK		
		Slow	Med	Fast	Soft	Med	Loud	Low	Mid	High	PS	SL	PL
M O V E	Preference	3	4	5	3	4	4	2	3	3	4	3	3
	Efficiency	3	4	5	3	4	4	2	3	2	4	3	2
	Self-Regulation	4-	4	5+	4-	4	4+	3	3	3	4+	3	3

Analyzing and Interpreting Scores

The MRS scoring example in Figure 10 examined the client's preferences, perceptual efficiency, and ability to self-regulate when engaged in movement in musical-play. The client scored a rating of "3" (exhibits musical response about half of the time) in the areas "preference" and "efficiency" in regard to slow tempo, soft dynamic range, middle pitch range, and staccato legato and primarily legato range of attack. The client also scored a rating of "4" (exhibits musical response often but not always) in the areas of "preference" and "efficiency" in regard to medium tempo and dynamic range and primarily staccato in range of attack. In addition, the client also scored a rating of "5" (consistently exhibits musical response) in the areas of "preference" and "efficiency" in regard to fast tempo range.

Chapter 5: Scale III: Musical Responsiveness Scale

In the area of self-regulation the client's rating scores indicated a "4" (exhibits response often but not always) in regards to medium tempo and dynamic range, a "3" (exhibits response about half of the time) pertaining to the entire range of pitch, and staccato and legato and primarily legato in range of attack. Finally, in the area of self-regulation the client scored "4-" (exhibits musical responses often but not always and dysregulates in a hyporeactive manner) in regard to slow tempo and soft dynamic, and "5+" (consistently exhibits musical responses and dysregulates in a hyperreactive manner) in regards to fast tempo.

Glossary

Adaption to musical-play: This term is taken from the Musical Emotional Assessment Rating Scale (MEARS) and refers to how the client times own musical-play in response to therapist; client follows what the therapist is doing as a play partner, but does not necessarily respond to specific musical elements. (Parallel play.)

Affect: An expression of emotion displayed through facial expression, motion, voice tone, hand gestures, laughter, and tears.

Attack (musical): The manner in which music is being performed, articulated, or expressed.

Affect synchrony: The matching of affective behavior between parent and child in which both engage in a continuous dialogue as they maintain a patterned relationship throughout play.

Circle of communication: A conversation (e.g., verbal, nonverbal, musical, etc.) in which two active participants respond to each other in a reciprocal and related manner. Circles of communication can occur through musical-play, gestures, spoken words, playing with objects, etc.

Clinical improvisation: A process in which the client and therapist spontaneously create music together to assess, treat, and evaluate.

Dynamic: The loudness or softness of a sound.

Follows: This term is taken from the Musical Cognitive/Perception Scale (MCPS) and refers to the client changing a musical element to match therapist; how client follows therapist in relation to specific musical elements.

Functional Emotional Assessment Scale (FEAS): A criterion-referenced instrument for children ranging in age from seven months through four years of age, designed to measure emotional functioning.

Hyperreactive: The client displays an exaggerated response (heightened sensitivity) to stimuli.

Hyporeactive: The client displays a low sensitivity to stimuli.

Initiates: This term is taken from the Musical Cognitive/Perception Scale (MCPS) and refers to how the client spontaneously manipulates a musical element in a meaningful way.

Melody: A sequence of two or more notes.

Mixed reactivity: The client exhibits both a low and high sensitivity to stimuli.

Motor planning: The ability to plan, sequence, and execute an action.

Musical affect: This term is taken from the Musical Emotional Assessment Rating Scale (MEARS) and refers to how the client responds affectively to musical-play.

Musical attention: This term is taken from the Musical Emotional Assessment Rating Scale (MEARS) and refers to how the client attends to musical-play.

Musical Cognitive/Perception Scale (MCPS): A criterion-referenced rating scale designed to examine the client's ability to react, focus, recall, follow, and initiate rhythm, melody, dynamics, phrase, and timbre.

Musical Emotional Assessment Rating Scale (MEARS): A criterion-referenced rating scale designed to examine the client's ability to musically attend, respond affectively, adapt/engage in parallel play, engage/participate in parallel-interactive play, and interrelate/engage in true interactive play.

Musical engagement: This term, taken from the Musical Emotional Assessment Rating Scale (MEARS), refers to the client using specific musical elements to match and engage therapist's music; client engages in therapist's music as cued, and not offering original musical ideas. (Parallel/interactive play.)

Glossary

Musical interrelatedness: This term, taken from the Musical Emotional Assessment Rating Scale (MEARS), refers to how the client contributes original musical ideas to engage in musical-play with therapist. (True interactive play.)

Musical-play: A form of interaction that involves two or more participants engaged in coactive music making.

Musical preference: This term is taken from the Musical Responsiveness Scale (MRS) and refers to the extent to which the client responds with positive affect in a particular media.

Musical Responsiveness Scale (MRS): A criterion-referenced rating scale designed to examine the client's overall responses and tendencies in musical-play (i.e., musical preferences, perceptual efficiency, and self-regulation).

Pitch: The quality of a sound based on the rate of vibrations; degree of highness or lowness of a tone.

Perceptual efficiency: This term is taken from the Musical Responsiveness Scale (MRS) and refers to the relative success that the client has in a musical medium when performing perceptual tasks.

Phrase (musical): A musical passage that contains a sequence of notes and rhythm within a musical meter.

Range in musical-play: The client's capacity to engage in related music making that includes a variety or a range of tempo, dynamics, and other expressive musical elements.

Reacts: This term is taken from the Musical Cognitive/Perception Scale (MCPS) and refers to the client responding affectively or behaviorally to a musical element and changes therein.

Recalls: This term is taken from the Musical Cognitive/Perception Scale (MCPS) and refers to the client recognizing or remembering repeated musical patterns by imitating, predicting, or ending therapist's music.

Reciprocal interactions: A mutual or cooperative interchange between two or more participants.

Rhythm: A recurring movement of sound, speech, or body movement consistently repeated at regularly timed intervals.

Self-regulation: The extent to which the client maintains attention, readiness, and availability for interaction.

Tempo: The speed (fast or slow) at which a piece of music is played.

Timbre: The quality of sounds outside of pitch, dynamics, or duration.

Two-way purposeful communication: Interactions that involve two or more participants engaging in a back-and-forth dialoguing (e.g., verbal, nonverbal, gestural, musical, etc.).

APPENDIX A IMCAP-ND FORMS

Intake Form

Rating Scales

Assessment/Evaluation Report

IMCAP-ND
INTAKE FORM

IMCAP-ND

INTAKE FORM

CONTACT INFORMATION

Client's Name:	**Chronological Age:**
Date of Intake:	**Grade:**
Date of Birth:	**Primary Language:**
School:	
Parent/Guardian:	
Employer:	**Work Phone:**
Cell/Mobile:	**Home Phone:**
Home Address:	**City:**
State:	**Zip Code:**
Email Address:	**Referred by:**

FAMILY HISTORY

Adopted?	**Age when adopted?**
Country of Birth:	
Name of Siblings:	**Date of Birth:**
1)	1)
2)	2)
3)	3)
4)	4)
Diagnosis:	**Diagnosing Doctor:**
Date of Diagnosis:	**Phone:**

INTERVENTION HISTORY

	Frequency	*Therapist*	*Phone*
Music Therapy			
DIR/Floortime			
ABA			
Psychology			
Occupational Therapy			
Play Therapy			
Physical Therapy			
Speech Therapy			
Other:			

MEDICAL HISTORY

Primary Physician: **Phone:**

Address: **City:**

State: **Zip Code:**

Email Address: **Phone:**

Pregnancy/Delivery   [ ] Normal   [ ] Complications

Describe:

Hospitalization?   [ ] Yes   [ ] No   How long?   At what age?

Describe medical conditions:

List medications:

List allergies:

DEVELOPMENTAL HISTORY

Age began sitting: **Age began talking:**

Age began crawling: **Age began toileting:**

Discuss concerns and observations:

LANGUAGE DEVELOPMENT

Does your child use language to meet needs?

If no, explain:

LANGUAGE DEVELOPMENT (CONT.)

Uses language to meet needs? [ ] Yes [ ] No

If no, explain:

Does your child primarily speak in: [ ] single words [ ] 2-3 word sentences [ ] complex sentences

Provide an example:

Is your child's language: [ ] easily understood [ ] usually understood

Does your child follow directions?

If yes: [ ] simple [ ] complex (more than 2 steps)

How does child express needs?

Explain:

Can child retell story in a logical order?

If yes, please explain:

COMMUNICATION

How does your child communicate with family and friends?

Please describe:

Can child comprehend and follow gestures during an interaction?

If yes, describe:

COMMUNICATION (CONT.)

Can your child comprehend and follow verbal instructions?

If yes, describe:

SENSORY

Is your child overly sensitive to: [ ] touch [ ] smell [ ] taste [ ] sounds

Comfortable w/ feel of clothes, fabrics, etc.?

Describe/Explain:

Comfortable being touched by others during play or social interactions?

Describe/Explain:

Comfortable in engaging in movement activities?

Describe/Explain:

SENSORY (CONT.)

Does child seek out or crave movement?

Describe/Explain:

Does child bump into things when navigating around the room?

Describe/Explain:

Is your child comfortable with sounds inside and outside the room?

Describe/Explain:

Is your child comfortable and able to manage/navigate in busy visual environments i.e., does your child get visually overstimulated?

Describe/Explain:

SOCIAL-EMOTIONAL

How does child respond to new situations and environments?

Describe/Explain:

SOCIAL-EMOTIONAL (CONT.)

Child prefers to play:	[ ] alone [ ] adults [ ] peers [ ] siblings
Initiates activities with peers?	
Describe/Explain:	
Child's passions:	
What special skills does your child have?	
What activities does your child like most?	
Child's strengths:	
Child's challenges:	

MUSICAL

Has your child had previous music therapy services? If so, where and for how long?	
Has your child taken music lessons before? If so, what instrument/s?	
Does your child display musical skills/abilities?	
Describe:	
Does your child listen to music?	
If so, what kind of music?	

MUSICAL (CONT.)

When and where does child frequently listen to music?

Describe:

Does child initiate musical activity?

[ ] singing   [ ] dancing   [ ] listening

[ ] playing instrument

[ ] parental involvement

[ ] sibling involvement

If yes, describe:

Does child sing along to music?

How does child respond when you join him/her in singing, playing instruments, and dancing?

Describe:

Are there musicians in the family?

Does your child have an interest in a particular instrument/s?

List:

OTHER INFORMATION

What would you like music therapy to do for your child?

Explain:

Please list any additional information that you feel is important:

PARENT COACHING

Have you ever participated in parent coaching? If yes, where and for how long?

Explain your experiences:

Would you like to participate in music-based coaching with your child? [ ] yes [ ] no

If no, Explain:

If yes, explain what you would like to achieve from parent coaching:

List your availability:

IMCAP-ND
RATING SCALES

IMCAP-ND

The Individual Music-Centered Assessment Profile for Neurodevelopmental Disorders

John A. Carpente, Ph.D., MT-BC, LCAT

Rating Forms

Scale I: Musical Emotional Assessment Rating Scale (MEARS)
Scale II: Musical Cognitive/Perception Scale (MCPS)
Scale III: Musical Responsiveness Scale (MRS)

Client's Name: _____ **Gender:** _____

Date of Birth: _____ **Chronological Age:** _____

Date of evaluation: _____ **Evaluator:** _____

Notes:
_____
_____
_____
_____
_____
_____
_____
_____
_____
_____
_____
_____
_____
_____
_____
_____
_____
_____

Copyright © 2013 by John A. Carpente. Not to be reproduced in whole or in part without written permission of the author. All rights reserved.

INSTRUCTIONS

SCALE I: MUSICAL EMOTIONAL ASSESSMENT RATING SCALE (MEARS)

Observe the target responses as they are exhibited during the session or segment thereof. Rate the frequency of the client's response (see frequency scale below). Then rate the support provided for the target response (see below) and indicate the media in which the client offered the target response with the initials I (Instrumental), V (Vocal), and/or M (Movement).

Frequency:
1 = exhibits musical response rarely if ever
2 = exhibits musical response occasionally
3 = exhibits musical response about half of the time
4 = exhibits musical response often but not always
5 = consistently exhibits musical response

Support:
1 = maximum (full physical)
2 = moderate (partial physical)
3 = mild support (visual)
4 = minimal (verbal)
5 = no support (independent)

Target Responses:

I. **MUSICAL ATTENTION:** How the client attends to musical-play.
  a) Focuses: attends to one or more aspects of therapist, music, or play.
  b) Maintains: sustains attention to one particular aspect of therapist, music, or play.
  c) Shares: attends to the same aspect as the therapist.
  d) Shifts: changes focus of attention as indicated by changes of therapist, music, or play.

II. **MUSICAL AFFECT:** How the client responds affectively to musical-play.
  e) Facial: expresses affect facially in response to therapist, music, or play.
  f) Prosody: expresses affect with voice in response to therapist, music, or play.
  g) Body: expresses affect through stationary movement in response to therapist, music, or play.
  h) Motion: expresses affect by moving toward or away from something in response to therapist, music, or play.

III. **ADAPTION TO MUSICAL-PLAY:** Client times own musical-play in response to therapist. Here, client follows what the therapist is doing as a play partner, but does not necessarily respond to specific musical elements. (Parallel play.)
  i) Joins: enters into musical-play as led by therapist.
  j) Adjusts: adapts own participation in musical-play as led by therapist.
  k) Takes turns: enters into alternating musical-play as led by therapist.
  l) Stops: stops musical-play when therapist stops.

IV. **MUSICAL ENGAGEMENT:** Client uses specific musical elements to match and engage therapist's music. Here, client is engaging in therapist's music as cued, and not offering original musical ideas. (Parallel/interactive play).
  m) Imitates: echos musical phrases as cued by therapist.
  n) Synchronizes: matches musical elements of therapist's music as cued by therapist.
  o) Predicts: anticipates recurring musical responses as cued by therapist.
  p) Ends: provides musical endings as cued by therapist.

V. **MUSICAL INTERRELATEDNESS:** Client contributes original musical ideas to engage in musical-play with therapist. (Interactive play.)
  q) Initiates: spontaneously begins a meaningful musical interaction with intent to invite therapist.
  r) Changes: spontaneously initiates meaningful, original changes in any musical element.
  s) Differentiates: takes role of soloist or accompanist using own musical material; contrasts own musical elements in relation to therapist.
  t) Assimilates: incorporates therapist's musical ideas into own original music.
  u) Connects: spontaneously bridges original musical material to a phrase and section.
  v) Interjects: inserts original ideas into musical spaces of therapist.
  w) Completes: uses own musical ideas to create closure to music.
  x) Leads/follows: independently initiates changes in leadership and followership roles with therapist.

Copyright © 2013 by John A. Carpente. Not to be reproduced in whole or in part without written permission of the author. All rights reserved.

SCALE I: MUSICAL EMOTIONAL ASSESSMENT RATING SCALE (MEARS)

Client: _____ Date: _____ Evaluator: _____

I. MUSICAL ATTENTION

	Frequency	Support	Media
a) Focuses			
b) Maintains			
c) Shares			
d) Shifts			
Totals/Avg.			

II. MUSICAL AFFECT

	Frequency	Support	Media
e) Facial			
f) Prosody			
g) Body			
h) Motion			
Totals/Avg.			

III. ADAPTION TO MUSICAL-PLAY

	Frequency	Support	Media
i) Joins			
j) Adjusts			
k) Takes Turns			
l) Stops			
Totals/Avg.			

IV. MUSICAL ENGAGEMENT

	Frequency	Support	Media
m) Imitates			
n) Synchronizes			
o) Predicts			
p) Ends			
Totals/Avg.			

V. MUSICAL INTERRELATEDNESS

	Frequency	Support	Media
q) Initiates			
r) Changes			
s) Differentiates			
t) Assimilates			
u) Connects			
v) Interjects			
w) Completes			
x) Leads/Follows			
Totals/Avg.			

Copyright © 2013 by John A. Carpente. Not to be reproduced in whole or in part without written permission of the author. All rights reserved.

INSTRUCTIONS

SCALE II: MUSICAL COGNITIVE/PERCEPTION SCALE (MCPS)

Observe the target responses as they are exhibited during the session or segment thereof. Indicate the media in which the client offered the target response with the initials I (Instrumental), V (Vocal), and/or M (Movement). Then rate the frequency of the client's response (see below). Thus, for example, "V/5" in the "focuses" row under "rhythm" column signifies that the client consistently attends to rhythm when singing.

Frequency:
1 = exhibits musical response rarely if ever
2 = exhibits musical response occasionally
3 = exhibits musical response about half of the time
4 = exhibits musical response often but not always
5 = consistently exhibits musical response

Target Responses:
I. **REACTS**: responds affectively or behaviorally to this musical element and changes therein.
II. **FOCUSES**: attends to this musical element as led by therapist.
III. **RECALLS**: recognizes or remembers repeated musical patterns by imitating, predicting or ending therapist's music.
IV. **FOLLOWS**: changes this musical element to match therapist; how client follows therapist in relation to specific musical elements.
V. **INITIATES**: spontaneously manipulates this musical element in a meaningful way.

SCALE III: MUSICAL RESPONSIVENESS SCALE (MRS)

After you have rated a session with Scales I and II, rate the overall preferences, perceptual efficiency, and self-regulation exhibited by the client throughout this session. Rate the overall tendencies of the client at the different ranges of tempo, dynamics, pitch, and attack using the frequency rating scale. When scoring self-regulation add a "+" for hyperreactive, or a "-" for hyporeactive, or a "±" for mixed reactivity. Thus, for example, "2 +" in the "fast tempo" row under "instrument" column signifies that the client is occasionally self-regulated and dysregulates in a hyperreactive manner during fast tempo music when engaged in instrument play.

Target Responses:
I. **PREFERENCES**: the extent to which the client responds with positive affect in this musical media.
II. **PERCEPTUAL EFFICIENCY**: the relative success the client has in this musical media when performing perceptual tasks.
III. **SELF-REGULATION**: the extent to which the client maintains attention and availability for interaction in this musical media.

Ranges:
a) **TEMPO**: slow (adagio) = 66–76 bpm; medium (andante) = 76–108 bpm; fast (allegro) = 120–168 bpm.
b) **DYNAMIC**: soft = piano; medium = mezzo-forte; loud = forte.
c) **PITCH**: low = C3–B3; mid-range = C4–B4; high = C5–B5.
d) **ATTACK**: PS = primarily staccato; SL = staccato and legato; PL= primarily legato.

Notes:
_____
_____
_____
_____
_____
_____

Copyright © 2013 by John A. Carpente. Not to be reproduced in whole or in part without written permission of the author. All rights reserved.

SCALE II: MUSICAL COGNITIVE/PERCEPTION SCALE (MCPS)

Client: _____ Date: _____ Evaluator: _____

	Rhythm	Melody	Dynamic	Phrase	Timbre	Total/Avg.
Reacts						
Focuses						
Recalls						
Follows						
Initiates						

SCALE III: MUSICAL RESPONSIVENESS SCALE (MRS)

		TEMPO RANGE			DYN. RANGE			PITCH RANGE			ATTACK		
		Slow	Med	Fast	Soft	Med	Loud	Low	Mid	High	PS	SL	PL
VOCAL	Preference												
	Efficiency												
	Self-Regulation												
INST	Preference												
	Efficiency												
	Self-Regulation												
MOVE	Preference												
	Efficiency												
	Self-Regulation												

Copyright © 2013 by John A. Carpente. Not to be reproduced in whole or in part without written permission of the author. All rights reserved.

CLINICAL OBSERVATIONS/LISTENING

NOTES:

NOTES:

MUSICAL THEMES

IMCAP-ND
ASSESSMENT/EVALUATION
REPORT

IMCAP-ND

Assessment/Evaluation Report

Client's Name:	Date of Birth:
Diagnosis:	Assessment Date:
Therapist:	Date of Report:

IMCAP-ND SCORES (MEARS)

Domain Areas	Frequency	Support	Media
Level I: Musical Attention			
Level II: Musical Affect			
Level III: Adaption to Musical-Play			
Level IV: Musical Engagement			
Level V: Musical Interrelatedness			

HISTORY AND BACKGROUND

GENERAL CLINICAL OBSERVATIONS AND MUSICAL EVENTS

Copyright © 2013 by John A. Carpente. All rights reserved.

DESCRIBE THE QUALITY OF MUSICAL RELATEDNESS/INTERACTIONS

DESCRIBE THE CLIENT'S RANGE PERTAINING TO MUSICAL RELATEDNESS

DESCRIBE THE CLIENT'S ABILITY TO INITIATE AND PLAY WITH THE INTENT TO RELATE

Copyright © 2013 by John A. Carpente. All rights reserved.

IMCAP-ND RESULTS (MUSICAL EMOTIONAL ASSESSMENT RATING SCALE)

I. Musical Attention

Musical attention deals with four areas pertaining to how the client attends to the various aspects of musical-play, including:

1) Focuses: attends to one or more aspects of therapist, music, or play.

2) Maintains: sustains attention to one particular aspect of therapist, music, or play.

3) Shares: attends to the same aspect as the therapist.

4) Shifts: changes focus of attention as indicated by changes of therapist, music, or play.

Strengths and challenges

II. Musical Affect

Musical affect deals with four areas pertaining to how the client responds affectively to musical-play, including:

1) Facial: expresses affect facially in response to therapist, music, or play.

2) Prosody: expresses affect with voice in response to therapist, music, or play.

3) Body: expresses affect through stationary movement in response to therapist, music, or play.

4) Motion: expresses affect by moving toward or away from something in response to therapist, music, or play.

Strengths and challenges

Copyright © 2013 by John A. Carpente. All rights reserved.

III. Adaption to Musical-Play

Adaption to musical-play deals with four areas pertaining to how the client times own musical-play in response to therapist, i.e., how client follows what the therapist is doing as a play partner, but does not necessarily respond to specific musical elements (parallel play), including:

1) Joins: enters into musical-play as led by therapist.

2) Adjusts: adapts own participation in musical-play as led by therapist.

3) Takes turns: enters into alternating musical-play as led by therapist.

4) Stops: stops musical-play when therapist stops.

Strengths and challenges

IV. Musical Engagement

Musical engagement deals with four areas pertaining to how the client uses specific musical elements to match and engage therapist's music i.e., how the client is engaging in therapist's music as cued, and not offering original musical ideas (parallel/interactive play), including:

1) Imitates: echos musical phrases as cued by therapist.

2) Synchronizes: matches musical elements of therapist's music as cued by therapist.

3) Predicts: anticipates recurring musical responses as cued by therapist.

4) Ends: provides musical endings as cued by therapist.

Strengths and challenges

V. Musical Interrelatedness

Musical interrelatedness deals with eight areas pertaining to how the client contributes original musical ideas to engage in musical-play with therapist (interactive play), including:

1) Initiates: spontaneously begins a meaningful musical interaction with intent to invite therapist.

2) Changes: spontaneously initiates meaningful, original changes in any musical element.

3) Differentiates: takes role of soloist or accompanist using own musical material; contrasts own musical elements in relation to therapist.

4) Assimilates: incorporates therapist's musical ideas into own original music.

5) Connects: spontaneously bridges original musical material to a phrase and section.

6) Interjects: inserts original ideas into musical spaces of therapist.

7) Completes: uses own musical ideas to create closure to music.

8) Leads/follows: independently initiates changes in leadership and followership roles with therapist.

Strengths and challenges

DESCRIPTION OF MUSICAL COGNITIVE/PERCEPTION IN MUSICAL-PLAY

DESCRIPTION OF OVERALL RESPONSIVENESS IN MUSICAL-PLAY

SUPPORTIVE INTERVENTIONS, INDIVIDUAL/MUSICAL DIFFERENCES, AND PREFERRED MEDIA

SUMMARY

Copyright © 2013 by John A. Carpente. All rights reserved.

EMERGING GOALS

1)
2)
3)
4)

INTERVENTION PLAN

RECOMMENDATIONS

_____   _____
Therapist's signature   Date

Copyright © 2013 by John A. Carpente. All rights reserved.

REFERENCES

Aigen, K. (2005). *Music-centered music therapy*. Gilsum, NH: Barcelona Publishers.

Alvin, J., & Warwick, A. (1991). *Music therapy for the autistic child* (2nd edition). Oxford: Oxford University Press.

American Psychiatry Association (APA) (2000). Diagnostic and statistical manual of mental disorders (4th ed.), Text revision. Washington, DC: Author.

Bruscia, K. (1987). *Improvisational models of music therapy*. Springfield, IL: Charles C. Thomas Publications.

Bruscia, K. (1998). *Defining music therapy*. Gilsum, NH: Barcelona Publishers.

Bryan, A. (1989). Autistic group case study. *British Journal of Music Therapy, 3,* (1), 16–21.

Carpente, J. (2009). *Contributions of Nordoff-Robbins music therapy within the Developmental, Individual Differences, Relationship (DIR®)-based Model in the treatment of children with autism: Four case studies*. Dissertation. Temple University. Ann Arbor: ProQuest/UMI, publication number AAT 3359621.

Carpente, J. (2011). *Addressing core features of autism: Integrating Nordoff-Robbins Music Therapy within the Developmental, Individual-Difference, Relationship-based (DIR®)/Floortime™ Model*. In A. Meadows (Ed.), *Developments in music therapy practice: Case study perspectives*. Gilsum, NH: Barcelona Publishers.

Carpente, J. (2012). DIR®/Floortime™: Implications for improvisational music therapy. In P. Kern & M. Humpal. *Early childhood music therapy and autism spectrum disorders: Developing potential in young children and their families*. Philadelphia, PA: Jessica Kingsley.

Cooper, Heron, & Heward (2007) *Applied behavioral analysis*. Saddle River: NJ: Pearson Publishers.

Feldman, R. (2007). On the origins of background emotions: From affect synchrony to symbolic expression. Emotion, *7,* 601 – 611.

Greenspan, S.I. (1992). *Infancy and early childhood: The practice of clinical assessment and intervention with emotional and developmental challenges.* Madison, CT: International Universities Press.

Greenspan, S.I., DeGangi, G., & Weider, S. (2001). *The functional emotional assessment scale (FEAS) for infancy and early childhood: Clinical and research application.* Bethesda, MD: Interdisciplinary Council on Developmental and Learning Disorders.

Greenspan, S.I., & Shanker, S. G. (2004). *The first idea: How symbols, language, and intelligence evolved from our primate ancestors to modern humans.* Cambridge, MA: Da Capo Lifelong Books.

Greenspan, S.I., & Weider, S. (2006a). *Engaging autism: Using the Floortime approach to help children relate, communicate, and think.* Cambridge, MA: Da Capo Lifelong Books.

Greenspan, S.I., & Weider, S. (2006b). *Infant and early childhood mental health: A comprehensive developmental approach to assessment and intervention.* New York, NY: American Psychiatric Association.

Honing, Henkjan (2012). "Without it no music: Beat induction as a fundamental musical trait." *Annals of the New York Academy of Sciences,* 1252: 85 – 91.

Interdisciplinary Council on Developmental and Learning Disorders (ICDL) (2005). *Diagnostic manual for infancy and early childhood.* Bethesda, MD: ICDL.

Levitin, D. (2006). *This is your brain on music: The science of a human obsession.* New York, NY: Penguin Group, Inc.

Nordoff, P., & Robbins, C. (2007). *Creative music therapy: A guide to fostering clinical musicianship.* Gilsum, NH: Barcelona Publishers.

Patel, A. D. (2010). *Music, language, and the brain.* New York: Oxford University Press.

Piaget, J. (1962). *Play, dreams and imitation in childhood.* New York: Norton.

Piaget, J. & Barbel, I. (1969). *The psychology of the child.* New York, NY: Basic Books.

Saperston, B. (1973). The use of music establishing communication with an autistic mentally retarded child. *Journal of Music Therapy, 10,* 184–188.

Tager-Flusberg, H. (1999). *Neurodevelopmental disorders.* Cambridge, Mass: MIT Press.

Wheeler, B., Shultis, C., & Polen, D. (2005). *Clinical training guide for the student music therapist.* Gilsum, NH: Barcelona Publisher.

Wigram, T. (2004). *Improvisation: Methods and techniques for music therapy clinicians, educators and students.* Phhiladelphia, PA: Jessica Kingsley Publishers.

Zero to Three: National Center for Clinical Infant Programs. (1994). *Diagnostic classification: 0 – 3. Diagnostic classification of mental health and developmental disorders of infancy and early childhood.* Arlington, VA: Author.

Zero to Three (2005). *Diagnostic classification of mental health and developmental disorders in infancy and early childhood.* (rev. ed.). Washington, DC: Zero to Three Press.

ABOUT THE AUTHOR

John A. Carpente, Ph.D., MT-BC, LCAT, Assistant Professor of Music and Music Therapy at Molloy College, is the founder and executive director of The Rebecca Center for Music Therapy, founding clinical director of the Center for Autism and Child Development, and owner of Developmental Music Health Services. He is also the founding music therapist and creator of the DIR®/Floortime™-based music therapy program at the Rebecca School in New York City where he participated in weekly supervision and case conferences with Dr. Stanley I. Greenspan, co-creator of the DIR®/Floortime™. He is also an instructor/clinical supervisor for the post-graduate Nordoff-Robbins Music Therapy advanced certification training at Molloy College.

Dr. Carpente has over fifteen years of clinical and supervisory experience working in a variety of settings as a clinician, clinical supervisor, and program director serving a wide range of client groups with developmental, neurological, and emotional challenges. A pioneer in DIR®/Floortime™-based music therapy, his clinical and research focus is on individuals with neurodevelopmental disorders and their families, parent coaching, assessment, and clinical supervision. He is currently the USA site manager for the TIME-A international music therapy and ASD research project, the largest randomized controlled trial on clinical interventions for autism to date.

Dr. Carpente has served on several boards and committees with special attention to autism and child development and his advocacy and consultation have resulted in the development of numerous first-time clinical and training programs in schools, clinics, community centers, and hospitals throughout Long Island and New York City.

Dr. Carpente has authored several book chapters and articles on the topic of developmental relationship-based music therapy and autism spectrum disorders, and has lectured on his work internationally and domestically.

Subject Index

A

adaption to musical-Play, 42, 113, 116

affect, 23, 85

analyzing andiInterpreting scores, 52, 68, 82

Angelman syndrome, 8

attack, 71, 72, 74, 75, 76, 78, 79, 82, 85

attention deficit- hyperactivity disorder

    ADHD, 8

autism spectrum disorders, 8, 121, 124

B

Bruscia, K., 8, 12–14, 50, 57, 60, 62, 64, 66, 72, 76, 79, 121

Bruscia's clinical techniques, 8

C

cause-and-effect

    relationships, 21, 44

circle of communication, 21, 50, 85

client's emotional life, 17

client's responses

    facial expressions, 7, 21, 23, 29, 31, 36, 85

    movements, 7, 12, 13, 18, 29, 30, 72

    visual spatial capacities, 7

    motor planning, 24, 44, 47, 61

    sequencing, 3, 7, 16, 24, 44, 61

    sensory sensitivities, 7

clinical improvisation, 13

clinical observations/listening, 38, 41, 44, 47

clinical techniques, 11, 14, 38, 41

    empathy, 20, 23, 28, 50

    structuring, 20, 28, 47,

    intimacy, 14, 28

    elicitation, 14, 23, 28

closing circle of communication, 22

communication, 13, 18, 21, 22, 27, 50, 85, 88, 123

continuous but constricted, 24, 25

    tempo, dynamic, 25

continuous flow, 21, 24, 25, 51, 73, 74

continuous through a range, 24, 26

    tempo, dynamic, 26

core features of neurodevelopmental disorders, 9

craving movement, 39

criteria of target responses, 35, 1, 55, 69

D

developmental, individual-differences, relationship-based, 16

differentiating, 13, 15, 23, 44, 51, 57, 64, 76

DIR®/Floortime™ Model, 13–15, 18, 35

Down's syndrome, 8

E

emotional lead, 16, 18, 20, 36, 37

evoking affective responses, 41

exaggerating, 14

extending, 15, 23, 38, 41, 43, 50, 60, 66, 72, 79

F

focus, 15, 36, 40, 52, 59

follow, 63

fragile-X syndrome, 8

fragmented and cyclical, 25

fragmented and intermittent (no consistent pattern), 25

Functional Emotional Assessment Scale, 85

Functional Emotional Developmental Levels, 35

G

genetic disorders, 8

Greenspan, S, 9, 16, 17, 21, 24, 35, 122

H

hand-over-hand

   HOH, 29, 33

hyper- or hyporeactive, 37

Hyperreactive, 85

Hyporeactive, 86

I

IMCAP-ND, 5, 12–15

   data collection, 6

imitating, 14, 20, 23, 38, 41, 50, 60, 61, 66, 72, 79, 87, 106

individual differences, 38, 41, 44, 47, 60

initiates, 4, 67, 86, 98, 104, 105, 107, 117

intensifying, 23, 44, 57, 64, 76

intentionality in musical-play, 26

interactive musical processes, 13

M

making space

   musical, 44, 47, 57, 62, 64, 76

maximum support

   full physical support, 33

MCPS, 2–5, 55, 85–87, 103, 106, 107

MEARS, 2–5, 28, 35, 51, 52, 85, 86, 103–105, 113, 115

medium support, 10, 30

   model, 30

   gesture, 30

   positional, 30

meeting perseverative behaviors, 20

meeting the client musically, 17

meeting the client's affect, 41

mild support, 30

   verbal cues, 30

mixed reactivity, 86

modeling, 15, 23, 30, 44, 47, 57, 62, 64, 76

Moderate support

   partial physical support, 32

moment-to-moment interactions, 11, 14, 15, 31

motor planning, 86

MRS, 2, 4, 5, 69, 70, 81, 82, 87, 103, 106, 107

music domain, 2, 35, 45, 48, 51

musical affect, 39, 40, 113, 115

musical attention, 36, 113, 115

Musical Cognition/Perception Scale, 55

musical contexts, 13, 16, 29, 37, 41, 42, 62

Musical Emotional Assessment Rating Scale, 10, 28, 35

musical emotional lead, ii, 17

musical engagement, 45, 46, 113, 116

musical environment, ii, 11, 18, 37

musical interrelatedness, 48, 49, 113, 117

musical media

   vocal, movement, instrument, 12

Musical Responsiveness Scale, 5, 69

musical tasks, 6

musical tendencies, 17, 18, 19, 22

musical-play, 12

   coactive music making, improvisation, 12

mutual music making, 26

N

Neurodevelopmental disorders

   autistic spectrum disorders, speech and language disorders, ADHD, fragile X, Down's Syndrome, genetic, 8 population-based, 8

nonmusical interventions, 8

Nordoff & Robbins, 13, 16, 18, 33

O

overall responsiveness

    MCPS, musical-play, 1, 2, 4, 69

P

parallel/interactive play, 45, 116

perseverative behaviors, 2, 11, 19, 58

preferences, 70, 71, 72, 87

procedural considerations, 15

procedural phases, 9, 11, 16, 17

    following client's lead, two-way purposeful musical-play, affect synchrony, 16, 17

procedures for supportive interventions

    verbal, visual, physical, 28

proprioceptive, 16

prosody, 41, 53

protocols and procedures, 3, 35, 55, 69

Q

quality of musical-play interactions, 24

R

range in musical-play, 26, 87

reacts, 4, 55, 56, 87, 107

recall, 61

reciprocating, 21

reciprocity, 21

redirect, 15, 30, 43

repeating, 15, 23, 37, 38, 41, 44, 47, 50, 57, 60, 62, 64, 66, 72, 76, 79

Rett syndrome, 8

rhythmic grounding, 14, 20, 23, 38, 41, 47, 50, 60, 62, 66, 72, 76, 79

Robbins, C., 13, 16, 17, 33, 121, 122, 124

S

Scale I: Musical Emotional Assessment Rating Scale, 5

scoring

    frequency, support provided, media, 3, 4, 35, 51, 52, 55, 67, 69, 81, 82

scoring instructions, 35, 55, 69

self-regulation, 4, 69, 77, 82, 107

sensory processing, 25, 61

session format

    client-led, 11

shaping, 14, 20, 23, 47, 50, 52, 66, 76

soliloquies, 15, 28

speech and language disorders, 8

spontaneous empathy, 13

synchronizing, 14, 19, 20, 23, 38, 41, 50, 60, 66, 72, 79

T

tactile, 7, 16, 36, 80

therapist's qualifications, 8

tonal centering, 14, 20, 23, 38, 41, 47, 50, 60, 62, 66, 72, 76, 79

V

vestibular, 7, 16, 80

W

Weider, S., 17, 21, 24, 25, 122

Williams syndrome, 8

Made in the USA
San Bernardino, CA
16 August 2014